Detox

The Lazy Person's Guide!

Detox

Belinda Viagas

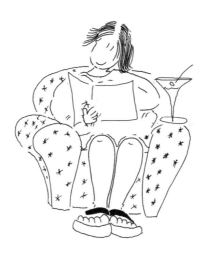

Newleaf

CONTENTS

INTRODUCTION

When I wrote the original Detox Diet book in 1991, I never imagined it would become a worldwide best seller, or be the inspiration for the zillion detox diets that would follow as practitioners and health writers published their own versions of the diet that worked best for them. The original little book has continued to sell because it is about a sound principle of natural healthcare – certainly not another faddy diet. It makes good common sense to spring-clean our body every so often, in much the same way as we spring-clean our homes, and the rest of our lives.

You detox because you know you need to. It is a way to clean out all those difficult bits that can be hard to reach, and leaves you with a body that feels cleaner, shinier, and more easy to use – a body that will work more effectively, rather than feeling bunged up or 'dusty'. A healthy body means that you can leave a host of health concerns by the wayside – including allergies, cellulite, the perils of slow digestion, a sluggish metabolism, and a weakened immune system.

The original Detox Diet was a comprehensive, month-long programme to cleanse and revitalise health, boost energy levels and banish allergies. Although based on foods, it also included a variety of support measures, from massage to meditation, that were optional extras to enhance and improve the work of the foods themselves. It captured everyone's interest, and now we are all much more familiar with the concepts of spring-cleaning our body as a route to improved health.

In this book, the principles remain the same, but the practice is made more accessible for everyone who doesn't have too much time to spare, or for whom juggling the many demands of modern life mean that everything, including health, must be squeezed into an already busy schedule. Those of us who feel these stresses are going to benefit most from whatever form of detox we can manage. A shorter detox also provides the perfect opportunity to top up the work of the original plan.

As our lives become ever busier, we need to prioritise our own healthcare so that we have a body that functions well and happily, and so that we have the energy we need to meet our commitments. This *Detox: The Lazy Person's Guide* looks at all the quick and easy ways that we can use foods and herbs and the principles of the detox and fit them into whatever time we have available to us.

This book, then, is for everyone who leads a busy life, and needs to juggle their own healthcare needs with a raft of other concerns. And you don't have to be lazy to follow its good advice!

The stresses we face today are like nothing we have known before. Beyond the pressures and time constraints of living a busy life and managing everything within it, we also need to deal with chemicals and pollutants in our food, our water, and the air we breathe on a daily basis. This all adds up to a complicated cocktail of substances that requires careful management lest it overwhelm us. These stresses can be compounded by our own genetic predispositions to certain health challenges. Yet in the midst of all these demands, our bodies still assert their own vitality and seek out optimum health.

We are amazingly competent, elegant and sophisticated organisms, with our own self-regulating mechanisms that will do their utmost to ensure maximum available energy and maximum 'wellness'. All we need to do is to allow these functions, and they will continue to do their best throughout our life. Sometimes the best thing we can do is just to get out of our own way, and give them the time and the space that is required for them to function at their best. And that is the very essence of detoxification.

To detox is to trust that your body's own innate intelligence and homoeostatic mechanisms will win through, and to give yourself the right internal environment for this to happen. It doesn't need to be done for a month at a time – this book shows you how to do it whenever and for as long as you choose; you don't even need to dedicate a special time to it, but can incorporate the basic principles into your existing lifestyle and let it work for you.

The key to detoxing your system is to make life as simple as possible for yourself, and for your body. In practice, this means no more confusing your body with chemicals and other additives when you can avoid it, and no more relying on your adrenal glands for energy when they are already fully taxed dealing with your other stress levels. It means supporting your body, rather than expecting it to work for you in the midst of ever-increasing challenges. Some foods, and some ways of eating, will naturally be easy for the body to deal with, and can help support the work of detoxification. By returning to a system that your body instinctively recognises, and is able to respond to, you activate the best possible self-healing processes.

Many of our everyday health complaints can be due to an

overload reaction that occurs when the body is no longer able to handle all the stresses it meets. Common symptoms such as endless colds, food intolerance, cold hands and feet, and low energy are often the first signs of a body that is in need of some help. Most of the people who consult me complain of a real lack of energy that overlies their other health concerns and, whether they also suffer with headaches or piles, they have all responded to a detox diet of some kind to return them to a level of general fitness and energy that is the key to all long-term good health. The best things about this book are that it is based on the experiences of lots of busy, busy people, and that it has been shown to work for them – fitting into their lifestyles and showing positive results.

When you cleanse the body effectively, not only is it easy to do, but you revitalise yourself – increasing your energy levels and creating a positive inner environment which means an end to weight fluctuations, an improved immune system, and the disappearance of minor and recurrent illnesses and ailments.

Detoxing is a dynamic technique which will give you a fitter body, a clearer mind, and will raise your spirits. With this book you can tailor your detox not only to fit your own unique needs, but also to fit your own personal timetable.

CHAPTER 1

WHY DETOX?

Everything has a season of rest: in the cyclic nature of life there is a time for activity, and a time for replenishment. The body does a remarkable job in terms of recognising, assimilating, digesting and releasing energy from our food, and then directing that to where it will be most useful, using it effectively, and processing and eliminating any by-products. It does all this before we even begin to think about picking up an arm, or moving from one foot to another! It does this every day, day in and day out: and it also needs to cope with a host of other concerns such as processing thoughts, responding to events, keeping us well and maintaining full energy. To rest the body is a powerful 'thank you' gift to ourselves that honours our own basic needs, and it is also a solid investment in our present and future wellbeing.

We naturally rest when we sleep each night, and let the body get on with all the routine housework, growth and renewal that we cannot do while we are awake. But we can do more than that. When we rest our digestion, we free up an enormous amount of energy that the body can use in whatever area it will be most needed. This energy is often used to tackle any stubborn health concerns; or it may be felt in terms of more available energy to get up and be active, making moving easier and leaving us with an overall awareness of increased vitality. Often healing occurs in reverse order, because the body tackles the most pressing problems first; so you may find that recent concerns are eased most quickly, while older or long-standing complaints take a little longer to resolve. This self-healing is a quite remarkable event, and one that we can all have access to, whenever we make the choice to free up the available energy through some form of detox.

The body naturally detoxifies by ridding itself of harmful substances in a continual process of cleansing. The ability to do this depends on our own vitality, and by aiding the body by following a detox plan, we not only help rid ourselves of a number of the toxins that can cause significant health problems, but we improve our individual health. The more we detox, the more able we are to do it better.

We are exposed to toxins from all quarters – in the foods we eat, the water we drink, the air we breathe, from our cooking utensils and dental fillings; and we also produce our own toxins through metabolic by-products, and from the role of bacteria in the gut. A good measure of full health is our ability to cleanse ourselves of these toxins and restore the system to full health. It's something that needs to be done regularly, and often.

Airborne pollutants such as the cadmium and lead from cigarette smoke can be involved in a range of disorders including anaemia, gut disturbances, hypertension, emphysema and osteoporosis. Lead is also to be found in canned foods, pesticide sprays, and many cooking pots. Mercury from dental fillings and vaccines can cause tremors, and there are strong links between metal toxicity and learning disorders and hyperactivity in children. The aluminium from our cooking pans, food wraps and antacid medication has been implicated in a variety of health challenges, including Alzheimer's disease.

Toxins that are produced within the body and not eliminated can cause real disruptions in the way the body works. It's rather like not taking out the rubbish, but just leaving it there in the corner of the rooms, and in the hallway. Over time, the piles build up, and your passage is impeded as you need to step over or around them in order to pass. A little longer and the piles get too big to allow you to pass, and by then it's starting to smell rather unpleasant too. You can't get in there to clean or hoover underneath it, and it attracts unwelcome visitors. In your body these can be infections and viruses. There are strong links between a build-up of these toxins and the range of auto-immune diseases such as rheumatoid arthritis, diabetes, and lupus, which cause both the immune system and the liver to come under increased pressure.

FOOD AS MEDICINE

We spend a lot of time and energy on our diet. In the history of humans, food wasn't always constantly available to us, and it is only in very recent times that many of us have not had to worry about getting enough to eat at all. Locked into our distant memory is an eating plan that is linked to the seasons and the natural availability of foods. It is quite a natural event to feast on some days, and fast on others. On a biochemical level, our bodies are still functioning in much the same way as our cave- and plain-dwelling forebears. We process foods in much the same way, recognise the same types of foods, and make the same types of decisions about them. The chemical treatments, additives, pesticides, fungicides, growth enhancers etc. that are routinely added to foods now are a very modern thing. Our bodies have not had the exposure to them to see whether their long-term effect will be harmless or not, and we certainly do not know how to respond to such a deluge of them.

Foods that the body does not recognise are treated as toxins and need to be eliminated from the system as quickly and as easily as possible. But this takes energy, and when we have more pressing needs for our energy, then this task can easily be on the body's 'to do' list for a very long time. Toxins also build up when we are eating well and wisely, but not giving time to the cleansing process.

Our bodies are remarkably resourceful; our primary brief, after all, is to stay alive. We can continue in the face of tremendous challenges and difficulties, and it is worthwhile doing all we can to make sure that we have all the vital resources that we need in order to maintain full health and wellbeing. Many of the degenerative changes we have come to accept as part of the ageing process may well be connected to our own lifestyle choices, and the lack of priority that we habitually give to our basic bodily needs. When we become busy and the needs of others, time constraints and a host of other things crowd in on us, it is common to put our own basic needs on a back burner. Good nutrition, sleep, exercise and self-care can become treats or chores, rather than basic everyday essentials. And yet everybody knows the secrets of good health, and they are remarkably simple. By prioritising health and making sure that we listen to and respond to our body's own basic needs we give ourselves a gift beyond measure; we allow the body to heal itself, and to walk forward into a future that is filled with the best health possibilities.

There may not always be things we can do to control the world 'out there'; we can, however, do a lot with our own inner resources. It is not just foods that we need to be concerned with; a polluted environment – whether immediately from second-hand cigarette smoke or carbon monoxide levels, or from wider environmental sources – can reduce the body's ability to get sufficient oxygen into the blood and remove carbon dioxide. This can also influence how well the body's organs are working, especially the liver, kidneys and digestive tract. Regular breathing exercises (see page 84) are an essential aid to maximise our lung capacity and ensure our system is not poisoned by elevated carbon dioxide levels. Used regularly, they can assist proper functioning of the whole body.

THE EFFECTS OF STRESS

Our response to stress is a wide and interesting one. We recognise as stress any number of things that challenge our ability to cope, and we can divide stress into two main categories – internal and external. When we see something that scares us (an external stress), we begin a process with the body that will enhance our ability to cope with it. We become more able to either stand and fight it, or to flee from it, as our body chemistry changes and energy is diverted away from digestion and the housekeeping work of the body's organs and towards muscular activity and heightened awareness. Just responding to this change can generate its own internal stress.

It doesn't have to be something that makes us frightened for our lives to generate this fight-or-flight effect – it can be seeing something scary on the television, or feeling insecure or uncomfortable in an unfamiliar situation. This means that the pressures of an interview or a trying business meeting, the demands of coping with young children, or even a night out going to see a film, can stimulate a system-wide response that needs to be dealt with.

We all know when we are feeling under this type of pressure. The symptoms of energy rushes, restlessness and irritability are our early warning signs that something is going on. Internal stress levels rise when this energy build-up is not discharged, but left to settle of its own accord – often just in time for us to respond to another wave of stress hormones.

When we are experiencing a flood of these hormones, it is not possible to digest food properly or fully, and that creates further internal stress.

The whole body is affected by stress. Some areas show signs of distress quite quickly; we soon notice tension in our own key spots – most often the shoulders, or sometimes the stomach. It may also affect us by highlighting a weak spot, such as the grumbling stomach that worriers experience, or the headaches that come from intense concentration and lack of sleep and fresh air. These are the signs that we can clearly see, but there is also a lot going on within the body that is not so visible; we do not usually see or feel the signs of internal stress right away.

The adrenal glands are two small and nowadays intensely overworked glands sitting on top of the kidneys. They are responsible for the release of the hormones that regulate our ability to deal with everything that we recognise to be a stress. The liver is a huge organ, sitting opposite the stomach on the right side of the rib cage, and it deals with filtering toxins out of the system, amongst other life-saving activities. Both the liver and the adrenal glands benefit from the time to recover that comes with a detox.

We are ideally suited to coping if we encounter stress – either internal or external – as an occasional thing. When we face it as an ongoing, relentless pressure every day then the effects can be ravaging. When the system is overloaded, it will deal with only the most important needs to keep us alive. The fight-or-flight stress response is a life-saver, and will always command our body's full attention. That means that while you will always be ready to run or fight to protect your life, you will not be achieving much in terms of absorbing nourishment from your food, or any of the less immediately vital but nevertheless essential work of maintenance and repair that is needed for tomorrow's health. As we spend more and more of our lives in this hyperexcited state, we expend more and more of our vital energy, robbing ourselves of our investment in our own future.

Tensions and perceived stress only increase, then, as we become less able to deal with them due to exhaustion of the vital hormones and other elements needed to face them (hormones are manufactured from the foods we eat, which need to be properly absorbed; B complex and other vitamins and minerals are needed to maintain the integrity and proper function of the nervous system – the way we send messages around the body – and these too come from the foods we eat ...). We can become caught in a vicious circle, as we again increase the stress we are experiencing by beginning to manifest the results of insufficient repair and maintenance, and proper assimilation, digestion and elimination. We can begin to see signs of malabsorption, an inability to relax, constant nervous irritation, skin complaints, a sluggish bowel, headaches, and eventually the possibility of chronic disease.

A number of our degenerative diseases can be directly linked to a history of overuse and overload. When the system is under this much pressure, something is likely to give, and there will need to be cutbacks. We begin to reject those things that require the most energy – like absorbing some energy-packed foods, or those that have complex or unfamiliar chemical structures. That means we add the weight of partially digested or assimilated foods to an already underachieving, overstressed digestion, and our body needs to switch its attention amongst an increasingly large number of highly pressing needs. So it is that we start to experience weight fluctuations, poor bowel health and all its associated problems such as headaches, increased pressure on the kidneys, indigestion, acid dyspepsia and stomach ulcers, as eating anything more becomes difficult.

We need to intervene and stop this degenerative cycle before its effects become too grave, and activate our own self-healing mode that will begin to reverse the negative effects of all these internal and external stresses. Simply spotting and stopping external stresses will do a lot, as will managing our own stress levels and activating our own Relaxation Response whenever stress appears. There are also things we can do with the foods we eat. These are our most immediate medicine, and one of the quickest ways to influence our own internal chemical environment. When we eliminate foods that are difficult to digest, or those which present too great a challenge, such as meals containing high levels of pesticides, preservatives and other chemical additives, then we relieve our dietary load and lift some of the pressure.

DIET AND STRESS

Few of us think of actively poisoning ourselves with the foods and drinks that we choose (with the possible exception of alcohol), but we have become quite used to regular consumption of a diet that is low in essential nutrients, high in fats and sugar, and that also contains low levels of potentially damaging additives and residues. Increasing numbers of us experience allergies to individual foods, or to food groups, and it seems obvious that there may be links to chemical pollutants and their still unknown effects within the body.

Following weight-reduction diets can induce its own stress. Having to count calories or watch everything you eat the whole time can result in depression, obsessive behaviour, or at the very least feelings of emotional deprivation. Your metabolic rate slows down too, when the amount you eat is restricted, so you end up with less energy and minimal weight loss overall. Once you start to eat 'normally' again, your slower metabolism has a hard time keeping up.

It's not only important *when* we eat; internal stress can also be caused by the food choices that we make. Some foods are easy for the body to process, and some require considerable effort and energy.

The work of this detox diet is not in reducing calories, or counting points, or any other weight-loss technique. If you need to lose weight, then you are likely to do so when you detox because your body will be rebalancing itself, healing itself and getting back to your own ideal weight. Healing yourself through the choices you make about foods and when and how you eat them is a great way to repair some of the damage caused by weight-loss regimes and a poor diet. It makes sense to avoid foods that have been denatured or chemically processed and altered out of recognition. It makes sense to have periods of rest and renewal in your busy life. It makes sense to learn more about your body's needs, and how best to meet them.

THE BENEFITS

The benefits of a detox plan will often be felt right away. Along with an immediate energy boost, existing health concerns begin to recede into the background, as the body is at last able to get on with its own healing and repair work.

To detox means that your whole body and mind will benefit, but it is a quite personal thing. Some people notice that the quality and softness of their skin improve very quickly; with others they first notice that their spots have cleared, or that rates of perspiration and body odour have positively changed. Whatever happens first is likely to be whatever your body needs to attend to most urgently, so there will be some difference between people, and even members of the same family may notice change in different places or at a different rate. What is certain, however, is that you will experience positive change.

Some of the most immediate positive benefits are often a clearer, softer skin, brighter eyes, and a general feeling of increased 'wellness'. This can go on to become much more specific as general health is improved and the whole system starts to pick up. The immune system gets a welcome boost, which means there is less likelihood of falling prey to viruses, and minor infections get cleared up very quickly. The lymphatic system supports this and makes sure that any localised water retention is removed from the system. Food intolerances quickly settle down or disappear altogether as digestion is strengthened and improved, and we become more able to get the energy that we need from the foods we eat. A less sluggish system means more energy is available to us whenever we need it. Mental clarity is increased, because the blood supply is clearer and able to deliver nutrients more effectively.

A body that is free of toxins can function more effectively, and a body that is working well feels good, has a slower ageing process, and has a greater energy resource to meet all our daily needs.

CHAPTER 2

HOW TO DETOX

To detox is to switch your body away from its jobs of coping with the stresses of the world, and of assimilating and digesting food – taking things in and processing them. It is to focus your body's energy instead on the work of eliminating, cleansing and renewal. Food is one of the best ways to influence which mode your body is in, and the clever use of foods will help you to switch painlessly from one way of working into another and back again, while ensuring you have all the energy that you need. Before you begin any detox, however short, make sure you read the section on Getting Started (page 32) to ensure that the transition is as positive and painless as possible.

WORKING WITH FOODS

The safest and easiest way to detox is not to fast, but to work wisely with foods and the way we eat them. There are different ways to approach a detox plan. We can look at the quantity of food that you eat, and seek to restore that to a more natural and beneficial level if it is a cause for concern. We can also work to moderate the amount, and control *when* we eat, in order to make life simpler for the digestion. This is also a consideration when we look at how long to spend on a detox. When time is at a premium, it is important to make sure that you get the maximum possible benefit from the amount of food you are eating, often in the shortest available time. In the next chapter we look at detox plans for just one day that will give you an instant health fillip, boost energy levels and help to relieve any digestive imbalance. There are also detox plans for two and three days, and one for a week – so there is no excuse not to begin one!

We can also look at the quality of the foods we eat. If we are choosing foods that are naturally rather than chemically grown, we are making life easier for both digestion and the natural filtration and detoxification work of the liver and kidneys. We also relieve this burden when we eat foods as close to their natural state as possible – without being processed, flavour-enhanced, or having a host of extra-added-goodness-knows-what. The way that you choose to detox will depend upon your own individual needs and the time you have available, so the detox plans in the next chapter are designed with very precise food choices to make sure you get optimum nutrition and the maximum benefits.

Not drinking too much with a meal will positively influence the ease with which we digest; and it is also important not to have any drink, or foods, that are too cold. Iced drinks and foods straight from the fridge are too much of a challenge to digestion, and use up valuable energy that could be used in processing the food and eliminating any waste products.

When we eat appropriately for our own health needs, and in tune with the seasons of the natural world, we are doing the most healthful thing we possibly can. Some foods are particularly good at enhancing the body's own elimination. Many fruits are high in water content and also rich in vitamins, so there is a double benefit.

When we can eat the skin of many fruits and vegetables because it is safe to do so, then we increase the amount of natural fibre in our diet and improve everything from peristalsis (the way food is moved through the gut) to bowel health. Some foods contain specific elements such as vitamins, minerals or enzymes that are especially useful to support the work of the key organs involved in a detox programme. Beetroot is a great tonic for the liver, for example, and pineapple and grapefruit help the gall bladder to release its store of fat-busting bile into the digestive process. Cruciferous vegetables are a valuable source of nutrients that will help support your body while you detox. These are all those vegetables whose leaves grow outwards in the shape of a four-pointed cross, and include the brassicas like cabbage, broccoli and kale.

Some everyday foods will be noticeable by their absence from all the detox plans. Wheat is a food we rely upon heavily – perhaps having toast or a wheat cereal for breakfast, a biscuit with coffee, a sandwich at lunchtime, and pasta for supper. Wheat has also been implicated in a range of health concerns, from sinus congestion to arthritis. Eliminating wheat from the diet and replacing it with other grains shows positive results for almost everyone who does it. It is a similar story with cow's dairy produce. It enters our diet by a variety of routes, and we can have many portions every day without trying too hard at all (milk in tea and coffee, a yoghurt snack, butter in a cheese sandwich, parmesan grated on to our pasta ...). Avoiding dairy produce is not too hard, because of the strong alternatives such as soya, and goat's and sheep's products, which are all easy to find and have none of the potential health concerns associated with cow's milk. If you experience sinus congestion, regular colds and flu, or any digestive complaints, a period away from cow's dairy produce would be a positive step.

How and *when* you eat are every bit as important as what. When you eat, and don't eat, at the best possible times for your body you maximise the benefits of the detox. Similarly, how you eat is vital to the success of any health-giving plan. It is important to be relaxed when you eat – we have already looked at how stress reduces our ability to digest food fully – but it is very common to have a business lunch, or eat in a noisy place filled with bright lights and primary colours, or when on the go. None of these things enables you to digest your food fully or well.

What we drink is also important to any detox programme. It is good practice to drink lots of good-quality still water, but not to have it too cold (avoid ice cubes if having within half an hour of food, lest you totally quench your digestive 'fire') or to drink too much with a meal. A small glass with food is usually sufficient to enhance digestion, and regular drinks throughout the day will help every part of you, from your kidneys to your skin.

ADDING HERBS

Herbs are a great addition to any detox plan as well as to everyday meals. There is often a rather thin dividing line between herbs and vegetables, and this can be a great pointer to one of the best ways of taking herbs – in a meal. Adding a little parsley to your meals can aid the work of the kidneys as well as helping to top up your iron levels (an important consideration for women), but do not eat too much, or have it during pregnancy. The top early leaves of nettles (picked before they sting!) make a wonderful blood cleanser that can easily be added to soups and salads.

Some herbs are traditionally associated with a detox plan, and these can be either added to the diet or taken as a separate herbal extract or tincture, or even in tablet or capsule form. Whenever possible aim to use fresh herbs, choosing them over dried or frozen; but when the fresh herb is not available, then take them as a supplement, close to or with a meal to ensure maximum absorption. Among the most useful herbs that will give good support during your detox are those listed below, and all will be available from your natural healthcare practitioner, or at your local health food shop. You don't need to take them for a detox plan to work, and you don't have to follow a detox plan for the herbs to work, but together they make a very positive and powerful combination.

- Silymarin or Silybanum – Milk Thistle. This is an incredible antioxidant that concentrates the regenerative powers of the liver in both the short and long term. You can start to see results the very next day when you begin taking it, and the benefits will continue. It is particularly useful if you drink a lot of alcohol and is very popular during the hangover season, because its fast action means it can relieve the symptoms or remove them altogether. You can get this in tablet form, or take a cup of tea made from the dried herb every day.

- Dandelion is a great aid to detoxification, because it is a natural diuretic which also supports the work of the liver and kidneys. In France, early dandelions are included with spring greens and eaten as a vegetable, but you can also take dandelion 'coffee' or root infusions: mix some dandelion in with a fresh juice, or take it as a herbal tincture (five drops in a little water twice a day).

■ Swedish bitters is a wonderful blend of herbs that all work together to enhance digestion, speed elimination and support the work of all the digestive organs. This is a tincture that can be taken before every meal, whether you are actively detoxing or not, and will greatly improve the way your body works. Take 5 ml in a little water before two meals every day for just a week, and you will feel the difference in terms of renewed vitality and improved skin tone.

■ Ginkgo biloba is the nut of the ginkgo tree and can be taken as a tea or in supplement form as a capsule or tablet. It radically improves blood flow to the kidneys, and is a powerful antioxidant and anti-inflammatory. Most often associated with improving mental clarity, it also has a place in a detox plan if water retention or associated concerns are a target for you.

When following any type of detox plan you will be focusing on supporting your body while it has a good clear-out. Take care when choosing anything to add to your diet, even beneficial supplements, to ensure that they are the highest possible quality. Look for organically grown or wild-crafted herbs, and check the ingredients on the labels of everything you intend to take. It needs to be free of artificial colourings or chemical alteratives.

FOLLOWING THE SEASONS

The basic idea of a detox is to make life simpler for your system, and eating what is seasonally available makes good sense for your body. It also enables you to get the maximum benefit from your detox. When you turn to the following chapters you will find detox plans for one day, two days, three days, and a week, and you will find options depending on the season. Essentially these are just cold-weather or warm-weather choices, although you can refine them still further by making sure that you pick foods that are seasonally available.

As we travel through the year, we see intense changes in the weather and in the world around us. We also see changes within our body. Spring sees the arrival of new shoots, and the delicious sweetness of baby vegetables alongside the bitter early saladings. This bitter is an excellent liver tonic, and any spring detox can capitalise on its natural availability to do the work the body most needs – to have a spring clean after the heavier winter fare. We can often feel our own energy lifting or rising at this time. Summer brings with it all the welcome warmth and light of the sun, and with it an abundance of vegetables and fruits, all ripe and ready for eating without the need for much preparation or cooking. This makes for a potentially very easy time on our digestion. With autumn come the harvest, the availability of fresh grains to provide us with an energy store for the approaching cold weather, and the berries - a last, rich, sweet boost of energy before the winter comes. Then the winter, when the world seems to stop growing, but all the energy is down below the ground in the roots and tubers that can provide us with so much good energy during the cold weather. This is the time to detox with the aid of clear soups, and to add grains to make sure we have the additional energy we need.

Warm weather is naturally favourable to the easiest types of detox – using fruits, juices, vegetables and salad meals. In the cold weather of winter you need warmth from your foods. This doesn't mean that it is impossible to detox: just that you need to tailor it specifically to avoid putting your system under additional strain. Follow the guidelines in each section, and pay particular attention to autumn and spring, when the seasons can take a long time to change: if it is snowing in April then follow the cold-weather advice, even if it is technically spring.

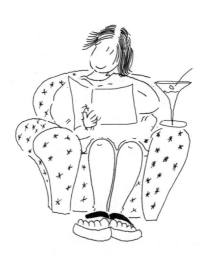

CHAPTER 3

GETTING STARTED

The time to begin your detox plan is yesterday. It doesn't matter whether you are following a detox that lasts for just one day, or a week, or a month: the work of the detox needs to begin the day before you start. Although there may be some practical details to attend to, like making sure you have enough good-quality, still water, or shopping for fresh food, the most important preparation is one that involves your body and mind.

When you think of a detox as a diet, the mental association you are likely to make will be with some form of deprivation. When you think instead about the idea of devoting some well-deserved time to a gift of replenishment and renewal for yourself, the prospect is quite different. Thinking ahead means you can change the whole tone of the experience by expecting to enjoy both the event and its benefits. Thinking ahead also lets you plan things so that you are able to avoid any potential pitfalls – a business lunch, or a children's party, would tax even the most committed detox plan!

You also need to prepare your body. The best possible start to a detox comes from having one of the preparation meals listed below as an early evening meal on the day before you officially start your detox. This way you make sure that your gut and your bowel are ready to forge ahead with the work of elimination, and will not be fazed by any dramatic shift of toxins into the system. You can assist this enormously by drinking a lot of good-quality, still water the evening before.

The body is an elegantly sophisticated system that is interconnected in a myriad ways. What you do or experience in one area will have effects everywhere else. The benefit of a food-based detox is that its effects will be felt throughout the system, and you can ensure that you do not risk expelling toxins from the tissues faster than the organs of elimination can work to get them out of the body. This can cause a build-up of toxicity in the blood and the lymphatic system, rather than curing it. When you use foods that are specifically chosen to enhance elimination, you know that you will be expelling things from your system and will be able to benefit immediately from the change. There are some wonderful support measures such as massage (page 87), breathing techniques (page 84) and exercise (page 88) that will reinforce the work of your eating plans, and you can also begin these the day before, or read up about them and be prepared to begin them straight away.

TARGETING YOUR DETOX

You can tailor your detox to fit your own individual health needs. Whether you follow a short or a quick-fix programme, you can be selective about the organs or areas of your health that you want to target, and there are also many ways to support their work on an everyday basis. In the following pages you will find advice for focusing your attention on your liver, kidneys, or digestion, along with some tips for making your gall-bladder a little happier (this is key to the digestion of fats), and relieving the pressure on your skin. Often the skin takes the pressure off a beleaguered bowel, and will show problems if there is sluggish elimination. It is unwise to concentrate exclusively on one area without professional advice, in case you unbalance the body and create more of a need for detoxification; but the following advice is a safe and supportive addition to your everyday diet.

Your liver performs great work, including producing bile to help breakdown fat, processing protein to make it safe, and metabolising alcohol and drugs. Its workload is astonishing and it carries out over 500 different functions, including regenerating itself. Eating a diet that is high in protein, drinking too much alcohol, or the regular use of some everyday drugs such as headache pills and antibiotics will mean your liver could do with a boost. Signs of a sluggish liver are not immediately apparent, but over time it can be responsible for nausea, migraines, allergic reactions and many other complaints.

Ease the pressure on your liver by reducing your everyday protein intake and including foods that are rich in vitamins C and E. These include all fresh vegetables, and dark green vegetables and wheat germ. Green tea is a powerful antioxidant that makes a very pleasant drink and will work to enhance the effects of the increased vitamins. Add raw beetroot to your diet as a regular treat – either fresh or as a fresh juice.

Your kidneys filter out toxins, waste products and excess sodium from your blood and eliminate them from your body in urine. They also produce an enzyme that regulates blood pressure. Too much salt in the diet (recommended maximum daily intake is 6 grams for men and 4 grams for women) is one of the major causes of strain on the kidneys. The second is drinking too little good-quality water or other neutral liquid, to keep the system fluid and reduce the risk of mineral salts forming stones and interrupting the work of the filtering mechanisms.

Make life easier for your kidneys by increasing the amount of good-quality, still water that you drink each day, but not drinking too much with a meal, or taking the drink too cold. Reduce your salt intake by taking salt off the table, and searching it out on the labels of any prepared foods that you buy. Increase the natural diuretics in your diet, including asparagus, parsley, dandelion and celery.

Digestion is a very big process that has distinct stages. The digestion of all starch begins in the mouth when you chew and mix your food with saliva. The process is mixed with acid in the stomach, and the liquid-like mass is passed through the digestive tract, or gut, in a fluid wave called peristalsis. Nutrients are absorbed in the small intestine, and waste material is concentrated in and passes out from the colon. A diet rich in fibre and water is needed to speed the movement of waste material.

The greatest ease to digestion will be regular detox days or short detox plans. In the meantime, increase the number of fresh fruits and vegetables that you have each day, and introduce whole grains – choose brown rice, whole-grain bread, barley, millet and quinoa as everyday alternatives. Consider taking some live yoghurt regularly to rebalance gut bacteria, or take a probiotic supplement.

Your skin is a vital organ that excretes water and salt and some of the waste products of metabolism, including uric acid, urea and ammonia. It is important to keep your pores open and allow your skin to breathe and take some of the eliminative strain off the kidneys and the digestive system.

Help your skin by keeping your bowels moving regularly (see

digestion, above) and by good breathing (see breathing exercises, page 84). Other measures include massage (page 87) or dry skin brushing (page 86). The skin responds very quickly to the presence of essential fatty acids in the diet, and it is important to pay attention to these. Reducing the saturated/animal fats in your diet and including some cold-pressed oil every day will show benefits very quickly.

The Detail

Whatever form of detox plan you choose from the following pages, these basic guidelines will get you started:

■ Prepare the day before by choosing one of the preparation meals below, drinking lots of water, and making sure you are feeling positively prepared to experience all the benefits.

■ Choose your detox plan, and make sure you do any necessary shopping to make it all possible.

■ Be prepared to eat – this is not a fast: the foods you eat and the way you eat them are important.

Dos and Don'ts

However long your detox plan, there are some basic rules that will help you to maximise the benefits:

■ Think natural. Choose foods that are free from additives, colourants, E-numbers, preservatives, synthetic flavours, etc.

■ Keep food fresh. Eat foods that are freshly grown wherever possible, rather than dried, canned, preserved or frozen.

■ Stick to the plan. Some things, like alcohol and tobacco won't be on any detox list, so make sure you exclude them and give your body a chance to fully appreciate the benefits of the detox.

■ Keep things simple. For your body this means avoiding drugs like caffeine and sugar, which lead to intense energy rushes and the resultant energy slumps, and can leave you dehydrated and sapped of energy.

■ Support your detox with any (or all) of the treats and treatments on pages 84–91. You can turn a regular detox into a truly healthful experience by expanding it to include all your senses.

■ Enjoy! Focus on the benefits, enjoy the freedom from your regular routine, and look forward to all the positive changes in terms of increased energy, softer skin, a stronger immune system, and relief from existing health concerns.

PREPARATION MEALS

The best possible meal to have the evening before a detox will depend on the season and your own personal likes and dislikes, so choose from the options below, or use these as a template to help guide you if making the meal yourself is not an option.

Brown Rice Salad
This is a wonderful, any-season meal that will prepare your digestive system and ready your bowel for however long a detox you have planned. Choose short-grain, brown rice to ensure

maximum fibre and maximum B-vitamins in your meal, and pick your own favourite selection of vegetables. During the colder weather, steam two or more of the vegetables to make digestion easier – during warm weather steam at least one.

INGREDIENTS

> 120 g of short-grain brown rice and 60 g barley
> Selection of seasonal vegetables – or favourite vegetables
> Salad leaves and fresh herbs of your choice
> Lemon juice
> Pinch of salt
> Good-quality oil such as cold-pressed olive or sunflower, or a
>   healthful blend such as Udo's Choice

DIRECTIONS

Rinse the rice and barley well and add to a pot of boiling water. Bring back to the boil and skim the surface. Cover and cook over a low heat for about 30–40 minutes or until grains are tender, but not mushy. Meanwhile, prepare your selection of vegetables for steaming, and chop the others finely and add to the prepared salad leaves. Steam the vegetables as close as possible to serving time. Combine the rice with the vegetables and the leaves and cover with a good squeeze of lemon juice, a small pinch of salt, and a generous dressing of oil. Mix and serve.

Lighter Supper

If you do not feel ready for the meal above, there are some lighter options. Choose from this list:

- Porridge thinned with a little soya milk and with a handful of raisins and a sprinkle of cinnamon added. A small amount of honey can be stirred in to taste.

- Warm dried fruit compote – made from a selection of dried fruits that have been soaked and then heated before serving. Take with a little live goat's or sheep's yoghurt.

- Fresh fruit.

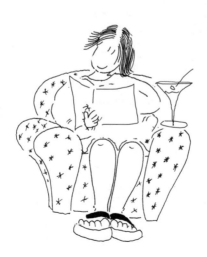

CHAPTER 4

YOUR DETOX PLANS

You can detox for anything from half a day to a month, depending on your own needs and time constraints. In this chapter you will find comprehensive plans for a One-day, Two-day, Four-day and Week-long Detox. You will also find a condensed version of the original month-long detox diet. The plans differ considerably, so read the directions for each detox before you start. The plans include the reasons why each type of detox will be so effective, and include clear directions for making the most of whatever time you have. Food lists and advice about when and how to eat are there to ensure that you get the absolute most from your time investment. These plans all focus on food, but the success of every detox will be maximised if you also undertake some of the support measures, exercises and treats that can be found on pages 84–91.

Although each detox plan is different, some elements will remain the same whichever one you choose. Certain foods and drinks will not be included:

coffee, tea and alcohol
cola and fizzy drinks
canned, packet, and ready-made foods
fried and fatty foods
wheat and dairy produce
animal protein

savoury snacks like crisps
chocolate
cakes, biscuits and pastries

Some foods are magic when it comes to reinforcing the work of your detox and encouraging your body to eliminate, and then supporting it in this process:

good-quality, still water
beetroot – a natural liver tonic
sprouted seeds and grains – high energy foods that are a rich source of enzymes, protein and nutrients
raw foods – high in energy and natural goodness
fresh fruit – a vitamin C boost that will enhance elimination
apples – reduce cholesterol levels, ease digestion and soothe a troubled or overtaxed gut
fresh ginger root – reduces wind and bloating, stimulates digestion and warms the whole system

Check each plan to see what specific foods are included or excluded, and also consider taking a multiple vitamin and mineral supplement (see page 61) if detoxing for longer than three days. You might also consider taking some of the herbal and other supplements outlined on pages 28–9 to strengthen or reinforce particular aspects of your health.

ONE-DAY DETOX

This is the perfect choice if you know you are going to have a day without too many commitments. Once you are used to the way that your body responds to a detox, you might choose to do this on a day when you have heavy commitments and need to redirect your inner resources towards managing the stress, and keeping your available energy high. To start with, though, especially if you have never followed a cleansing routine before, this is an ideal introduction. It is incredibly simple to follow, and produces instant results.

Begin, if possible, the evening before, and have one of the recommended evening meals. (See Getting Started, page 32.) This will set the inner stage for your detox and ensure that your digestion is working smoothly and well. One of the aims of a detox is to aid elimination, and it is important to keep the bowel clear so that you can eliminate in the most natural way – with a bowel movement.

You will be actively setting your body into elimination mode for the next 24 hours, and it is important to focus all your energy on this aim. The recommendations for what to eat, and what not to eat, are outlined below, but you would also benefit from some of the support measures such as breathing exercises (see page 84), and some gentle massage (see page 87). You can do this for yourself, or consult a professional massage therapist.

Food Choices

One of the simplest ways to focus your body's energy on elimination is to provide it with food that will keep the bowel moving, and provide energy for you to get on and do things, but which will rest or simplify digestion. Eating just one kind of food at regular intervals throughout the day, and drinking plenty of water, means that your body can easily assimilate and process the food – it can prepare for it because it knows what will be coming next, and it will not tax your energy or divert it from the process of elimination.

If the stomach has only one kind of food on which to work, which takes only a short time to digest, your energy can then be conserved, having obtained the maximum nutrition from the food you have eaten. This is excellent in the short term, and encourages elimination to a much greater extent than a balanced diet. This is especially good if there is any history of digestive upset, or if you have simply been eating too rich a diet recently.

Choosing a food to eat for your one-day detox from the list below is mainly a matter of taste, although health concerns can also influence your decision. If your primary need is for good levels of freely available energy, then grapes would be a good choice. They are high in natural fruit sugar and will provide a reliable source of energy throughout the day. Grapes are also a good choice if you have any rheumatic concerns. If you have any history of tummy upsets or digestive disturbance, choose apples. These are high in pectin and also malic acid, which stimulates gastric secretions and acts as a gentle soother for the gut. Dark red cherries and peaches are both good in season, and can be useful if you suffer with gout or any type of congestive problem. Ugli fruit is one of the most eliminative choices.

Fruits to choose from: apples, pears, pomegranates, grapes, ripe dark cherries, ugli fruit. In high summer you can also choose peaches. Do not eat anything else.

- Choose one fruit only. Make sure that you buy much, much more than you think you will want to eat (you may be surprised at your own appetite!) You are likely to eat much more than you might suppose, because you will only be eating that one fruit.

■   During winter, spend the day eating one of these fruits that is gently cooked in a minimum of water, and serve warm. The best choices for this are apples, pears, grapes or cherries.

■   Eat as much of the one fruit that you have chosen, as often as you like throughout the day.

■   Do not eat after 8 pm.

Your plan for the day will also involve drinking lots of good-quality, still water. You can filter your water, or choose a bottled mineral water. Do not drink anything else.

■   You will need to have a glass of water at least every 2 hours. Aim to have at least 1.5 litres over the course of the day.

■   In the winter you should drink hot water to keep yourself warm.

■   You can add a slice of lime to the water to aid gentle elimination.

■   Do not drink with your fruit – wait about twenty minutes.

That's it. It is as simple as that. For one day, you will pick a fruit and eat as much of that one fruit as you want to – either snacking on it as and when you feel like it, or sticking to regular 'meal' times and eating three times. You will also drink lots and lots and lots of water to flush out your system. And that's all you will have. This is not a recipe for one meal – it is your whole intake for the entire day.

You will have finished your detox when you have your last meal of fruit at around 8 pm, and will then be able to have only drinks of hot or cold water until bedtime. This will let your stomach rest completely and continue the work of cleansing while you prepare for bed, and while you are asleep.

The signs of a good detox are often felt the next morning, when you will be able to expect to wake refreshed after a good night's sleep, feeling more energetic and ready for the day ahead. You may also experience a big bowel movement, if you did not have an extra one the day before.

You can continue the good work of your day's detox in your choice of breakfast – have a fruit breakfast, and plan to break your detox properly at lunch-time. Have some more of your detox fruit and add one other fruit to it, so that you begin to prepare your system for having a little more variety.

You will find that you are already into a second day of cleansing almost without realising it.

On the following pages you will find plans for longer and longer detox – you can spend as long on it as you feel you will benefit from, so long as you stick to the directions. This one-day detox is an ideal introduction to cleansing and revitalising your body in this way, and you can follow it whenever you feel inclined. Most people would benefit from doing this as often as once a week. Just think of the difference it would make to your system! This is also a perfect way to 'top up' the effects of a longer detox that you might do only once a month, or even once a year.

TWO-DAY DETOX

This is a lovely way to really get in touch with your body's own needs, and will fit neatly into a weekend. Taking a little longer enables you to maximise the benefits of your detox, and give your system a thorough rest, as well as an opportunity to prioritise elimination. It is important that you follow the directions carefully, and include some of the support measures on pages 84–91 to ensure that you maximise your efforts and get an optimal return for your investment in this process.

Over the course of the next forty-eight hours you will be giving your digestive system an almost complete rest, and enabling your body to get on with any overdue or routine maintenance work that may have had to be sidelined because of your busy schedule or stressful lifestyle events.

Plan ahead to make sure that you have all that you need to enable your two-day detox to be a success, and that you really have made the time for this to happen. Choose a weekend or another time when you will be able to relax a lot, and follow your own timetable – resting when you choose to, and being able to get out or get on and do things when you feel bursts of energy. Try to minimise commitments, so that you can focus on your own internal health and wellbeing, and concentrate on your own inner relationship with yourself.

Internal mental preparation not only means you are more likely to succeed in following your detox plan, but also makes you more likely to maximise the benefits you obtain by doing it. Be prepared to not eat some foods, and to change your routine; and be prepared also to look and feel great, as you give your body the help it needs to maintain optimum energy and vitality.

Begin if possible the day before, by checking through your obligations to make certain that this is the best time for you to do your two-day detox; checking that you have the necessary ingredients to make your detox a success; and by having one of the starter meals on pages 37–9.

Food Choices

The foods you choose from on your two-day or weekend detox have been carefully selected to ensure that you maintain your blood sugar levels and will therefore have a constant supply of energy. They also have a high water content, to assist elimination through your skin, bowel and kidneys, and you will see the benefits quite quickly in terms of improved skin texture and quality. Most importantly, you will be taking them in a form that means your digestive system will be able to process and assimilate the nutrients with the greatest ease. This is also a very quick way of losing a few pounds in weight and ridding your body of any water it may be storing.

During the warmer months, you will be having your food in juice form to maximise your intake of energy and essential nutrients, but still keep digestive work and effort to a minimum. Juices play an important role in any healthcare plan and can focus digestive energy on elimination, as well as providing a revitalising rest for the whole system.

Juicing is the quickest way to prepare a healthy and nutritious meal that is easy to absorb and very tasty. It can transform humble ingredients into a real treat. Beyond your two-day detox, juices are invaluable for times when it is difficult to have a full meal – like at breakfast time when the prospect of eating can be a challenge, or when time is pressing. They also make a good meal substitute, or a healthy snack.

You can juice just about anything – with the exception of

especially pungent foods like garlic which can be an enormous challenge to drink and which will leave their mark in your juicer for ever. Juicers are now readily available, and you can choose one to suit your pocket. As a general rule the more expensive the machine the greater the strength of the motor, which means that each piece of fruit is likely to render more juice, and that the machine will last longer.

For the next two days, you will be having combined juices made from a carefully chosen blend of vegetables and fruits. Alternate these snack meals with drinks of water throughout the day to ensure you maintain the energy levels you need.

Vegetable and fruit choices for your 2-day, warm-weather detox: Carrots, celery, lettuce, beetroot, courgettes, parsley, apricots, pineapple, apples, pears, grapefruit, lemon, lime

- Aim to choose as varied a selection of juices as possible. Make sure that you buy much more than you think you will want because juicing makes food seem to disappear. Experiment with combinations that work best for you, and check out some of the juice recipes on page 50.

- All the food must be raw, and as fresh as possible. Some exceptions are possible: raw beetroot can be difficult to find unless you grow some yourself. A very good-quality organic juice is available in bottles from most health food shops. Freshly squeezed pineapple and grapefruit juices can also be found in the chilled cabinet of your local supermarket. Other than these two, do not be tempted to buy other juices: juice them yourself for maximum nutrients and a real blast of vitamin C.

- Take at least a small glass of juice every 3–4 hours, and intersperse this with at least a tall glass of good-quality water.

- Hold the juice in your mouth and 'chew' it a little to make sure it is well blended before you swallow each mouthful. This ensures that it is mixed with the salivary enzymes necessary for complete digestion.

- Have your final juice by 8 pm.

- During winter, you will need to have healthful broths or special soups rather than juices. When the weather is cold, juices for more than half a day would simply be too challenging for most constitutions, and could cause digestive concerns rather than solving them. Choose from the above ingredients and follow the recipes on page 50 carefully.

The success of your plan for the two-day detox will also rely upon your drinking lots of good-quality, still water. You can filter your water, or choose a bottled mineral water. Do not drink anything else. You can, though, have your water hot or boiled, and can add a slice of lemon to it, or in the colder weather a cardamom seed.

- You will need to have a glass of water at least every 2 hours. Aim to have at least 1.5 litres over the course of the day.

- In the winter make sure that much of your intake is hot in order to keep yourself warm.

- You can add a slice of lemon or lime to the water to aid gentle elimination.

■ Do not drink with your juice or soup – wait about 20 minutes. If you find the juice is too thick or is too much on your stomach, then dilute it 50:50 with water.

Juice Recipes

Some favourite, and very beneficial, juice combinations include:

2 carrots, 1 apple and 1 pear.

$\frac{1}{2}$ pineapple, 1 apple and a small slice of lemon

2 parts pineapple and 1 part grapefruit

2 carrots, 1 stick celery, 1 small head of lettuce, splash of beetroot juice and 1 pear

1 courgette, 2 sticks celery, 1 sprig parsley, a few lettuce leaves

Broth and Soup

Potassium broth

1 small swede

1 parsnip

1 slice pumpkin

2 carrots, trimmed or peeled if using chemically grown

1 onion

5 or 6 small potatoes

Roughly chop the swede, parsnip and pumpkin and one of the carrots. Place in a saucepan containing 500 ml water and bring to the boil. Cook for 5 minutes. Transfer to a blender and work till smooth. Return to the pan and add the remaining carrot, chopped, the finely chopped onion and the potatoes. Add another 300–500 ml of water and cook for 10–15 minutes or until the vegetable pieces are soft.

An alternative is an oriental-type clear soup, made by simmering together any of your selection of vegetables with the addition of some thinly shredded fresh ginger root, some finely sliced scallions or spring onions, and a large shot of tamari (wheat-free Soya sauce).

When making broth or soup for your 2-day detox, make one large pot at the beginning of the day and you can then vary the recipe for the second day.

Finishing Your Detox

You will have finished this detox when you have your last juice (or soup) at around 8 pm on day 2, and will then be able to have only drinks of hot or cold water until bedtime. For this last juice, stir in 2 large spoonfuls of live goat's or sheep's yoghurt (or stir it into your soup). This will help to prepare your gut for more solid food, and introduce a healthy probiotic balance to enhance your ability to cope with it.

Be careful when breaking your detox the next day. Make sure that you do not overtax your digestion after its rejuvenating fillip. Have a cup of warm water with a slice of lime or lemon in it upon rising, and then make breakfast one of the fruits that you have been juicing over the past two days. This will be a gentle introduction to a familiar but solid food. During the morning, continue to drink lots of water, and if you feel hungry snack on fruit. Make your lunch that day a salad meal, again relying heavily on foods that you have been juicing, perhaps with the introduction of one or two other vegetables, and leave having a cooked meal until evening.

FOUR-DAY DETOX

This is a great way to treat yourself to a long weekend of cleansing, or it can be done midweek to make sure that you have all the available energy you need to meet your commitments. Being able to take some time over this plan means that you are able to widen your choice of foods, which means you are less likely to become bored, and also that you are certain to ensure a rich intake of vitamins and other essential nutrients.

The key to the success of your four-day detox is in the quality of the foods you choose, and the way that you eat them. In the shorter plans you will have been concentrating on making things happen very quickly – supercharging your eliminative routes and organs and making them stand to attention. With this slightly longer detox, the focus will be on making life simple for your digestion, partly through food choice and partly also by supplying mega-doses of excellent nutrition in ways that your body can easily access.

Taking four days to do this means there is ample time for you to include some of the exercises and support measures, such as breathing techniques and massage (see pages 84–91), that can transform a short detox into a truly pleasurable and energetically profitable experience.

Food Choices
Throughout the next four days you will be eating food in its most natural state, enabling you full nutritional access and optimising enzyme activity with every meal you eat. The choice of foods you

can eat is very broad, and only those which you should avoid have been listed below. It is very important that you choose only the very best-quality foods, and seek out naturally or organically grown produce wherever possible. Otherwise you will need to peel most of the food you eat, and will lose much of its nutrient value, as well as losing some of the cleansing benefit that comes from eating pure food that is without the taint of pesticide residue or the potential internal challenge of chemical cocktails.

Starting on day one of your four-day detox – although if possible you should have prepared for this the evening before with one of the preparation suppers on page 37–9 – you will follow the same basic timetable throughout each day. It is important that you do not fast, but eat as much as your appetite leads you to, and eat and drink at regular intervals.

All of the food you eat will be raw, and your choice of fruits and vegetables is as wide as your local shops will allow. Ideally your day would start with a cold or hot drink of good-quality water, to which you can add a slice of lemon or lime. Breakfast can be one piece or a selection of different fruits, and you can also make your own choice of fruit for morning snacks. Your main meals, and all afternoon and evening snacks, will be salad-based, and so virgin olive oil, sunflower oil or a good blend such as Udo's Choice can be included, along with a squeeze of lemon or lime juice and a host of herbs to make a tasty salad dressing that is also packed with nutrients. Alternatively, you can dress your salad with a little live goat's or sheep's yoghurt. Other than that, the only foods you will be eating will be raw fruits and vegetables. You can eat them singly, or in whatever combinations appeal to you. You can make a huge bowl of salad and dress it differently at each meal or snack time, or you can chop up a range of vegetables and have them as crudités. Try putting your salad ingredients into the blender until they are shredded really fine and appreciating the different texture and sense of satisfaction this gives you.

Also included in this detox are any and all sprouts. This is the only type of grain you will be eating, and it opens up a whole world of energy and taste for you to explore. You can eat sunflower or pumpkin seed sprouts, mung or navy bean sprouts, and barley and wheat grass sprouts. You will find chickpeas, alfalfa, lentil, corn and green pea sprouts in most health food shops, and many supermarkets also carry a range. You can sprout an amazingly wide range of foods quite easily by keeping them in a jar by your kitchen sink and rinsing them regularly with warm water. Most sprouts will appear within three to five days. They generally have greater nutrient activity than all other raw foods, and provide protein, roughage and enzymes to improve digestion, stimulate detoxification and elimination and break down fats.

Some fruits and vegetables are excluded from this detox because they do not aid the work of internal cleansing, or because of their specific effects. Tomatoes for example are very acidic, and can be too challenging on a short detox such as this. Oranges can have a congestive effect on the liver and also need to be avoided. Also avoid or limit spinach, sorrel, mushrooms, coconut, rhubarb and plums.

Throughout your four days you will need to keep drinking large amounts of good-quality water. Try not to drink with a meal, but bear in mind that we can often misread thirst as hunger, so if you find yourself wanting a snack, have a glass of water, and see if you are still hungry for food after ten minutes or so. You can drink your water hot or cold; and also included in this detox are both green tea, which is high in antioxidants and will aid elimination through the bowel, and a limited range of herbal teas. It is recommended that you make these up to quite a weak infusion, and you can drink them hot, warm or cold. Over the next few days you will find your palate becomes much more discerning, and you will appreciate and be able to respond fully to the more subtle flavours. Choose from peppermint, linden or lime flower, rosehip and hibiscus, or fennel.

During the colder weather, you will need to take a hot drink of water, weak herbal tea or green tea with each meal and snack. You may also need to include some cooked grains rather than the sprouts – choose short-grain brown rice, basmati rice, barley or millet. Cook up a small amount to have warm with each meal and also include some fresh root ginger with each meal. You choice of herbal teas will also change for the colder weather, so select any of the following: cardamom, red zinger blend, chamomile, licorice root, rosemary or sage.

Each day:

- make sure that you eat – don't be tempted to skip a snack or a meal. Start the day with breakfast.

- Drink lots of warm or cold drinks from the recommended lists.

- Aim to have as much variety as possible in your selection of fruits and vegetables.

- Do not eat after 8 pm.

Preparing for a Wider Diet

After four days of following this detox plan, your body will have settled into a nice routine and should be feeling very happy! Introduce yourself to cooked foods again slowly, to maximise the benefits of your detox and make for a smooth transition.

On the fifth day of your detox, have a fruit breakfast, and snack on any fruits throughout the morning. At lunchtime have a salad, as you will have become used to, but include with it some cooked food. Let your desire lead you. If you fancy a jacket potato, or some protein, or would rather have some warm rice or other cooked grain, stop for just a moment and imagine that food already in your system. If your tummy feels fine, then go ahead and eat it. Make your afternoon snacks vegetable-based, and make sure your evening meal is also salad-based, but includes some cooked food also. On the next day you will be able to include more cooked foods, and a wider range of foods, if you feel like eating them; but let your body guide you, and take your time over returning to your usual diet.

Recipes for salad meals and for the next, week-long detox can be found in the recipes chapter on page 65.

WEEK-LONG DETOX

A week is a wonderful time to detox for. It lets you settle into the good habit, and removes much of the stress of having to think about what you are choosing and eating as you relax into your new routine. You can follow this week-long plan just once every now and then, or as an annual treat, or four times a year with the changing of the seasons. Whenever you can fit it in to your schedule you will begin to reap the benefits from day one, when energy levels will begin to even out, and you will start to feel better, clearer and more energised.

If this is your first introduction to a longer detox plan, you might like to include some of the herbal and vitamin supplements suggested on pages 27 and 61. These and the non-food measures will form a valuable part of your detox plan.

To detox for a week means really making it a part of your life, and the health benefits and energy changes you will experience mean that your life is never likely to be the same again.

Food Choices

A careful choice of foods will mean that you will be able to carry on with your normal, everyday schedule of commitments while ensuring that you have all the energy that you need to meet them – as well as releasing additional energy for inner healing and replenishing. The luxury of a whole week of time means that you will be able to pass through different modes of elimination and still maintain a clear view of the detox.

As with every detox, the work begins the evening before you start, and having one of the preparation meals outlined on pages 37–9 will set up your body to begin eliminating in the best possible way.

Days 1 and 2 are the same. You will be eating a combination of raw foods, but taking care not to mix fruits and vegetables together. Choose any vegetables that you like, with the exception of peppers, tomatoes and spinach, and make these form the bulk of your diet. You can eat them any way you choose – as a salad with one of the salad dressings listed below, or as crudités, alone or in combination with other vegetables. You can shred them, slice them thinly, eat them whole or grate them. Only peel them where you have to, or if the food has not been naturally or organically grown (pesticide levels in the skins of chemically grown produce are too high). Your choice of fruits is also extremely wide, with the exception of berries, rhubarb, coconut and melons. As with the vegetables, choose as wide a selection of fruits as you will enjoy, and eat them singly or mix them together. You could make a large bowl of mixed fruit salad each day and help yourself to it whenever you want, or you might enjoy savouring the deliciousness of individual fruit.

Dress your salads with either virgin olive or sunflower oil, or a good blend such as Udo's Choice, and a squeeze of lemon or lime juice. Avoid salt, but maximise flavour by adding any selection of fresh herbs with the exception of sorrel. You can also dress your fruit or vegetable salads with a small portion of live goat's or sheep's yoghurt.

Aim to drink at least 2 litres of good-quality, still water, and you can take this hot, with a slice of lime, or cold. Also drink either green tea, or choose from the following herbal teas and drink throughout the day: rosemary, sage, saffron, licorice, linden or lime flower, and chamomile are all good choices. Make them quite weak, and do not have more than two cups of any one herbal tea in any one day.

- Make sure that you eat lots: don't starve yourself or fast.

- Eat at least three meals each day and make sure you have breakfast.

■ Do not drink with your meals; wait for 20 minutes after eating before you have anything to drink, unless you are taking a supplement which needs to be taken with your meal – in which case take it with a small glass of water.

■ Do not eat after 8 pm.

On Day 3 you will be limiting your intake to vegetables only, following the guidelines for days 1 and 2: just eliminate the fruit. Make sure that you keep eating lots, and have breakfast, although it might seem a little strange to be eating something savoury in the morning. You will be providing energy to meet your body's needs, so do not be tempted to skip this vital meal. Remember to keep up your intake of water, and for today you can also include some cardamom seeds – add one to each cup of hot water or weak herbal tea that you have. This will help warm your digestion and keep your system moving.

Day 4 will be a juice day. Read the guidelines on pages 48–9 , but limit your choice of ingredients so that you are having mainly vegetables and only one fruit. Pick papaya, apples, pears or grapes. You can have as much juice as you like throughout the day. Dilute each small glass of juice with at least one tablespoon of good-quality, still water, but add more if you prefer, and have a glass of water in between each juice. Aim to be having something at least every two hours, but more frequently if you feel the desire or the need.

On Day 5 you repeat the plans for Day 3, with the addition of whichever fruit you chose to include in your plan yesterday. After a day of juicing your system will want to start back to solid food quite slowly, so make breakfast a single fruit or vegetable – papaya, apple or pear are good, or carrot or celery: but follow your own wants. Close your eyes and imagine the food in your tummy before you go ahead and eat it. Be sure to chew the food well. Wait about one hour after your first solid food, and then have another piece of the same fruit or vegetable along with something else. Continue to broaden your selection of food throughout the day, and make sure to keep drinking lots of good-quality, still water.

Days 6 and 7 follow the plans for days 1 and 2, but you can also add a small portion of goat's or sheep's cheese if you like. This can be crumbled into a salad or eaten in very small slices or pieces on its own. Its sharp taste will wake up your system, and introduce valuable nutrients, as well as preparing you to widen your diet as you come to the end of your detox week. It is especially important that you continue to drink lots of good-quality, still water during this time, particularly if you are adding the cheese to your diet.

At the end of this long a plan, it is a good idea to take at least one or two days to reintroduce a full range of foods. Start slowly, following some of the advice contained in the earlier, shorter detox plans. Make sure that you do not impose too great a stress on your system by indulging what you think your taste buds might like, but include one new food, food group or type of preparation with each meal. Close your eyes and imagine how a food will feel before you actually eat it, and keep drinking lots of good-quality, still water!

THE ORIGINAL DETOX DIET

This is a month-long programme that is designed for you to follow once, preferably in the warmer weather, although you can do it during winter if you follow the guidelines about keeping yourself warm.

It is split into three stages. Stage I is a transition from your normal, everyday diet and is a gentle introduction to the detox plan. It takes three days. Stage II is the main detox that you will be following for the majority of the month and is where most of the replenishing and rejuvenating work of the detox will be done. Stage III covers the final four days and serves to reintroduce you to a regular diet again.

This longer programme allows for a wealth of change as your body switches into a strongly eliminative mode, and you will see weight loss, the disappearance of old health concerns and challenges, a reduction in cellulite and fat deposits, the eradication of allergies and an increase in how good you look and how good you feel. It is the most radical, and totally natural, health tool that you could have, and it is totally specific and completely personalised. That means that your body will be deciding upon what work needs to be done, will be setting its own timing for the healing to occur, and will be able to repair and replenish just where it is most needed.

It is recommended that you take a multi-vitamin and mineral supplement while you follow this month-long programme. Let your choice be informed – be guided by your natural healthcare practitioner, or research this yourself. The quality of this supplement will be as important to you over the next month as the quality of the food you are eating, so choose a product that is free from additives and preservatives, that does not contain arbitrary packing material or unrecognisable substances, and make sure it does not contain additives, preservatives, colourings or sugar. You can find supplements that are wheat- and dairy-free, hypo-allergenic and these will positively enhance your detox.

Stage I

For the first three days of your month-long programme:

■ Drink 2 litres of water each day

■ Eat three meals a day

■ Start each day with a cup of hot water with a slice of lime or lemon in it

■ Do not eat after 8 pm.

Have fruit for breakfast – either fresh or rehydrated dried fruit – and mix it with any raw seeds, e.g. sunflower, sesame, pumpkin; and some live goat's or sheep's yoghurt.

For lunch and dinner, have rice and steamed vegetables and salad. Choose short-grain, brown rice mixed half-and-half with basmati rice. Dress your salads with virgin olive or sunflower oil, or a good blend such as Udo's Choice, and lime or lemon juice.

Drink water, or any selection of herbal teas, throughout the day.

Stage II

This lasts for days 4 to 25 of your month-long detox, and forms the major part of this plan.

■ Start each day with a drink of hot water with a slice of lime or lemon added

■ Drink at least 2 litres of water each day

■ Eat at least three meals – breakfast is a MUST

■ Do not drink with meals or for 20 minutes afterwards

■ Every day make sure that you have:

1 portion raw beetroot or a small glass of beetroot juice
1 small piece of fresh root ginger
1 serving of seaweed or sea vegetable
1 portion of sprouted nuts, grains or seeds
1 multi-vitamin and mineral supplement.

Breakfast each day needs to be fruit, but not oranges, coconut or rhubarb. You can choose any other fruit, or combination of fruits, and also have any raw seeds, e.g. poppy, sesame, anise, caraway; and some live goat's or sheep's yoghurt.

Lunch and dinner will combine any of the following:
short-grain, brown rice mixed half-and-half with basmati rice
any sprouted beans, seeds or grains
any fresh herbs except sorrel and rocket
any raw vegetables except mushrooms, tomatoes and spinach
any seaweeds or sea vegetables
1 portion of goat's or sheep's cheese per day
1 portion of goat's or sheep's yoghurt per day
freshly squeezed lime or lemon juice with virgin olive, sunflower or sesame seed oils, or a good blend such as Udo's Choice
snacks include any raw, unsalted nuts and seeds
drinks include any herbal teas
any fresh fruit juice except orange, diluted with at least 1 tablespoon of water per small glass
any freshly extracted vegetable juice diluted half-and-half with water, but not tomato or spinach

Stage III

This is the final few days of your month-long programme and begins your transition to a wider diet again. It is essential that you do not rush, but allow yourself to make this change slowly and carefully. If at any time you feel you are pushing yourself too quickly, go back to the previous day's directions and stay at that level until you feel ready to move on. During this stage you keep to the main detox plan you have been following in Stage II, but make the following additions:

On the first day of this stage (day 26 of this programme), include one steamed vegetable with one of your meals.

On the second day of this stage (day 27), include one steamed vegetable with two meals.

On the third day (day 28), have two meals containing a steamed vegetable and also include some protein; choose from tofu (bean curd) or fish, and steam cook them. If you are choosing tofu, add either a dash of tamari (wheat-free soya sauce) or a pinch of crushed cumin and one of crushed turmeric to the dish to aid digestion.

On the fourth day (day 29), have a soup or purée made from more than one vegetable at one of your meals. The rest of the day you should stick to the Stage II plan.

On the final day (day 30), have a stir-fry dish with one meal – use olive or sunflower oil to cook in, and choose any selection of vegetables and either tofu or a small amount of fish or fowl.

Once your detox is complete, you will be able to follow your taste buds and let your body's own true needs guide you towards those foods which will be best for you.

CHAPTER 5

RECIPES

Making sure that the quality of your food is as good as possible will maximise the effects of your detox. Whenever possible choose foods that are naturally grown, in season, and really fresh. Follow the guidelines in your main detox plan for food lists, and then sample some of these recipe ideas to see just how delicious a detox can be. You can use some of these recipes even when you are not following a detox plan – just work them into your regular diet for a healthy alternative.

SALAD DRESSINGS

Basic salad dressing

2 parts extra-virgin olive oil or a good blend such as Udo's Choice (especially good in the winter)
$\frac{1}{2}$ part lemon or lime juice

VARIATIONS

Add a handful of fresh basil leaves, a crushed clove of garlic and two or three sprigs of parsley for a strong-tasting, healthful, herby blend.

Add finely chopped coriander leaf (not the stems) and choose lime juice for a silky, smooth and very settling dressing.

Add pumpkin seeds and a handful of parsley and blend until smooth. This tasty dressing is excellent for supporting elimination through the bladder and is also good for the lungs.

Yoghurt Dressing

Mix live goat's or sheep's yoghurt with freshly chopped herbs – try mint and basil, shredded watercress, or dill.

Cucumber Raita

1 cup live goat's or sheep's yoghurt

1 small cucumber, peeled and finely diced

3 scallions or spring onions, finely chopped (the green and the white parts)

$\frac{1}{4}$ teaspoon powdered ginger

$\frac{1}{8}$ teaspoon ground turmeric

bunch of fresh coriander, finely chopped

Combine all the ingredients together and leave to stand for about 5 minutes before serving to allow the flavours to fully infuse.

Ginger Relish

1 large fresh ginger root

$1\frac{1}{2}$ cups water

1 large cooking apple

grated rind of 1 lemon and 1 lime

$\frac{1}{2}$ teaspoon dried ginger powder

Peel and grate the ginger. Place in a pan with the water, chopped apple, peel and ginger powder. Cook over a medium heat for 15–20 minutes or until the apple dissolves and the mixture becomes thick. This is an excellent and tasty treat to stimulate digestion. Keep it in the fridge and have in small amounts with a dry salad.

Peanut and Ginger Dressing

2 tablespoons peanuts
1 teaspoon fresh root ginger
$\frac{1}{4}$ cup water
1 tablespoon tamari (wheat-free soya sauce)
1 teaspoon tahini (sesame seed paste)

Peel and chop or crush the ginger root. Combine with the rest of the ingredients in a food processor and blend until smooth.

SALADS

Broccoli and Ginger

1 cup broccoli florets
2 tablespoons chopped almonds
1 spring onion, finely chopped
2.5 cm piece fresh root ginger, peeled and finely chopped
1 tablespoon olive oil
juice of $\frac{1}{2}$ lime

Separate the broccoli into small sprigs, and place in a bowl with the almonds and chopped spring onion and ginger. Pour the oil and lime juice over the salad and mix well together.

Carrot and Cumin

    1 large carrot, grated
    1 teaspoon crushed cumin
    1 teaspoon lime juice
    1 teaspoon grated fresh ginger root

Mix all the ingredients together in a bowl, and leave to stand for 1 hour to let the carrot become infused with all the flavours. You can also make this by slicing the carrots very thinly lengthwise and leaving a little of the leaf on.

Chicory and Fennel with Coriander Dressing

    1 head chicory, finely chopped
    1 fennel bulb, finely chopped
    1 lettuce heart, finely chopped
    1 bunch coriander leaves, shredded
    olive oil, lime juice and crushed coriander to dress

Place the chicory, fennel and lettuce in a salad bowl, and cover with the dressing ingredients. Mix and leave to stand for at least 5 minutes before serving.

Chayote with Basil and Sesame Seeds

    1 chayote, diced
    1 tablespoon sesame or sunflower seeds

FOR THE DRESSING
1 tablespoon olive oil
1 tablespoon lime or lemon juice
1 tablespoon finely chopped basil
1 crushed clove of garlic
1 shredded carrot to garnish

Combine the chayote with the seeds in a bowl. Blend the ingredients for the dressing and pour it over, mixing well. Strew with the shredded carrot.

Artichoke Coleslaw
1 cup Jerusalem artichokes
2 carrots, grated
2 spring onions, finely sliced

FOR THE DRESSING
5 tablespoons live goat's or sheep's yoghurt
1 tablespoon lemon juice
pinch of celery seeds or celery leaf
1 tablespoon sunflower seeds

Scrub the artichokes and grate them. Add to the carrot and onion in a bowl. Combine the ingredients for the dressing and pour over the salad. Mix well and serve straight away.

Marinated Kebabs

selection of young fresh vegetables, e.g.:

12 baby onions or shallots
12 broccoli florets
12 mangetout
12 baby carrots or strips of larger carrots

MARINADE

8 tablespoons olive oil
2 tablespoons lime or lemon juice
2 tablespoons freshly chopped mixed herbs
1 clove garlic, crushed
1 teaspoon crushed cumin
1 teaspoon freshly squeezed ginger juice

Place all the prepared vegetables in a dish. Combine the ingredients for the marinade and pour over the vegetables. Leave them to stand overnight or for at least a few hours. Thread onto long bamboo skewers and sprinkle with finely chopped parsley.

Carrot and Raisin Salad

3 large carrots
$\frac{1}{4}$ cup of raisins
$\frac{1}{2}$ cup of boiling water
1 teaspoon lime juice
1 large bunch fresh dill
8–10 sweet grapes
$\frac{1}{4}$ cup sunflower or virgin olive oil or a blend such as Udo's Choice

Pour the boiled water over the raisins and leave to soak for about 10 minutes. Wash and grate the carrots. Peel them for a slightly sweeter dish (and certainly peel them if they have been chemically grown). Mix up the dressing by combining the dill, lime juice and oil. Drain the raisins and stir them into the carrots along with the quartered grapes. Dress and eat straight away.

Courgettes with Carrots and Nasturtium Flowers

2 large carrots, grated
2 courgettes, grated
25 g sunflower seeds
25 g pumpkin seeds
nasturtium flowers
basil leaves

FOR THE DRESSING
2 tablespoons sunflower oil
1 teaspoon lemon juice
1 teaspoon freshly squeezed ginger juice

Place the carrots and courgettes in a serving bowl with the seeds. Combine the ingredients for the dressing and add to the bowl. Mix well. Arrange the nasturtium flowers on top and sprinkle with whole basil leaves.

Avocado Spread

    1 large avocado
    1 tablespoon lime juice
    1 small clove garlic
    1 small bunch fresh coriander
    grind of black pepper

Open, peel and discard the stone from the avocado. Peel and chop the clove of garlic, and sort through the coriander, picking off the leaves and the thinner tops of the stems, discarding the rest. Mix all ingredients together by mashing or blending in a food processor.

This recipe can also be made into a salad dressing by increasing the lime juice to 4 tablespoons, adding 4 tablespoons of water, and including the whole of the coriander.

SOUPS

Summer Borscht

    1 grated carrot
    1 onion, finely chopped
    450 g grated raw beetroot
    2 pints water
    juice of 1 lemon
    2 tablespoons live goat's or sheep's yoghurt
    1 tablespoon finely chopped coriander
    1 tablespoon finely chopped parsley

Place the prepared carrot, onion and beetroot in a blender

with the water and lemon juice, and blend until smooth. Serve in individual bowls with the yoghurt and herbs.

Creamed Almond Soup

    50 g ground almonds
    1 teaspoon coriander seeds
    1 tablespoon freshly shredded basil
    1 teaspoon fresh thyme
    300 ml live goat's or sheep's yoghurt
    1.2 litres water
    1 teaspoon lemon rind
    1 tablespoon almond flakes to garnish

Put the ground almonds, coriander seeds, basil and thyme into the blender with the yoghurt and water. Work until thoroughly blended. Add the lemon rind and stand for half an hour. Work the mixture again, then transfer to individual serving bowls and garnish with the almond flakes.

SWEET THINGS

Seed and Apple Cake

    175 g sunflower seeds
    175 g sesame seeds
    150 g dates, diced
    3 apples, grated
    1 teaspoon allspice
    few fresh strawberries or 1 more apple, sliced, to decorate

Grind the seeds and place in a mixing bowl. Add the dates, apples and allspice and mix well together. Place into an oblong tin and chill well until firm before serving. Turn out and decorate with strawberries or apple slices.

Cheesecake

225 g live goat's or sheep's yoghurt
125 g fresh apricots, stoned and chopped
50 g sesame seeds
50 g sunflower seeds
25 g almonds

Strain the yoghurt through muslin overnight into a bowl to get a really thick, creamy filling, or buy Greek yoghurt which is already really thick and creamy. Mix the yoghurt with the apricots. Crush the seeds and almonds and press in an even layer to make the base, then pour the yoghurt mixture on top. Refrigerate for at least an hour before serving.

Top with Apricot and Vanilla Purée

450 g fresh apricots, stoned and quartered
$\frac{1}{4}$ pint fresh apple juice
$\frac{1}{4}$ pint water
1 vanilla pod

Soak the apricots in the apple juice and water with the vanilla pod for at least 4 hours. Remove the pod and place the apricots and liquid into a blender. Work to a purée and chill lightly before serving.

Kiwi and Ginger Salad

2 kiwi fruit
3 apples
small bunch green grapes
1 tablespoon freshly squeezed ginger juice
4 tablespoons fresh apple juice

Peel and slice the kiwi fruit and slice the apples thinly. Place in a serving bowl with the grapes. Stir gently to combine, then cover with the ginger juice and apple juice. Serve right away, with a little live goat's or sheep's yoghurt.

Peach Surprise

4 large, ripe peaches
300 ml white grape juice

Peel and slice the peaches and place them in a ceramic or glass dish that holds them snugly. Pour over the grape juice and leave to stand for 2–3 hours so that the flavours can develop before serving.

COOKED MEALS

Steamed Vegetable Medley

1 small swede
2 carrots, trimmed or peeled if you use chemically grown
1 courgette, trimmed
handful of peas

Slice the swede, carrots and courgette and place in a steamer over a pan of boiling water. Cook with a lid on for about 3 minutes, then add the peas. Cook for a further 2–3 minutes or until the vegetables are just tender. Serve with a teaspoon of good oil and just a drop or two of lime or lemon juice and a few torn basil leaves.

Low Water Cooking

This is a good alternative to steaming, and any vegetables can be cooked this way to maximise flavour and minimise any nutrient loss.

Choose a selection of mixed vegetables, e.g. carrots, celery, peas and courgette
    5–6 large lettuce leaves
    2 tablespoons water

Chop vegetables into small pieces or thin slices. Line a saucepan with the rinsed lettuce leaves. Add the chopped or sliced vegetables and the water. Bring to the boil watching carefully, because you will hardly see the water level, then cover with a tight fitting lid and turn the heat down straight away. Simmer gently for 3–5 minutes.

Baked Squash

    1 butternut squash
    $\frac{1}{2}$ teaspoon crushed cumin
    $\frac{1}{4}$ teaspoon crushed turmeric
    1 tablespoon good oil
    $\frac{1}{4}$ teaspoon honey

Slice the squash in half down its length and remove the seeds. Place on a tray in a hot oven for 15 minutes. Take out and sprinkle with the cumin and turmeric, then return to the oven to cook for a further 10 minutes or until soft. Remove from the tray and scoop out the flesh, mashing it with the oil and honey.

Nori Rolls

1 cup of cooked rice (choose a mix of half-and-half short-grain brown rice and basmati)

3 leaves of nori

1 small courgette, trimmed

Slice the courgette into thin strips. Place a nori leaf on a plate and cover one end of it with a small, flattened strip of rice. Arrange some courgette strips along the length of the rice, and cover with another small strip of rice. Roll the nori up over the rice so that the courgette appears in the middle. Wet the end of the leaf to seal it and leave to stand for a few minutes. Slice across the rolled-up lengths and serve with salad or steamed vegetables.

Spicy Sprouts

1 cup of mixed sprouted seeds, peas, beans or grains. A good mix is 2 parts mung to 1 part chickpea, or fenugreek and alfalfa

1 tablespoon sunflower oil

$\frac{1}{2}$ teaspoon crushed turmeric

$\frac{1}{4}$ teaspoon crushed cumin

2 tablespoons lemon juice

Wash the sprouts well. Heat the oil in a pan, and add the turmeric and cumin. Add the sprouts and cook for 3–4 minutes over a medium to high heat until they soften. Add the lemon juice and eat straight away.

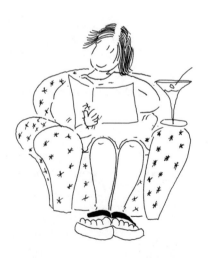

CHAPTER 6

BACK-UP INFORMATION

The information provided in the previous chapters is sufficient to enable you to detox safely and effectively on your own. Every one of us is different, though, and so our own experience will be influenced by our own situation, our individual constitutional strengths and challenges, and where we are in our lives. There are some themes that come up again and again, and some questions that I am almost always asked – beginning with what you can expect to experience physically while following a detox plan of any length.

Women will experience particular changes while undertaking any detox plan. Our cycles change with the seasons, and in response to stress levels and many other life events. Following a detox plan for even a day around mid-cycle or ovulation will have a positive impact upon the quality of the next menstrual period. This is a natural time for the body to detoxify, and whatever work is done mid-cycle relieves the pressure when the period comes. Many women find that menstrual difficulties and irregularities disappear if they follow a regular detox of up to three days each month when they ovulate.

Because the body's acidity is likely to change while following any detox plan of more than three days, you may notice some symptoms of thrush. These will disappear if you continue with your detox, or you can take specific steps to address them. They are best treated in consultation with your natural healthcare practitioner, but in the short term large amounts of live yoghurt taken with food and applied locally, the addition of a capful of cider vinegar to bath water for regular use, and the elimination from the diet of sugar (including fruit), wheat and yeasts will usually prove quickly effective.

Most often people start to notice the most obvious things first, namely the increase in sustainable energy, and the disappearance of all the peaks and troughs that can be caused by an overdependence of stimulants and sugar in the regular diet. A close second is an improvement in skin quality and texture – most people start to shine quite quickly – and a general feeling of overall wellbeing.

There are always questions about potatoes – people always ask whether they can eat them, and the answer is an unqualified 'yes' – cleaned and grated or shredded they can be included in any of the detox plans that permit an unspecified selection of vegetables. The taste and consistency of raw potato can be a new experience, but small amounts of it are a useful addition to any detox plan.

The reasons for all the choices and exclusions in the detox plans are well founded. Wheat, for instance, is excluded from all the plans because its effect on the body is quite acidic, and one of the aims of a detox is to make the body more alkaline. Wheat is also a very common allergen, mainly because we eat so much of it. We can quite happily rely on it almost exclusively as the only grain in our diet. Think about a normal day when you might have toast or a wheat cereal for breakfast, a mid-morning pastry, a sandwich at lunch, a biscuit in the afternoon, and pasta for supper. That makes for five portions of wheat a day, and this is not an uncommon day for many of us. Wheat has been associated with a variety of health concerns, from excess mucus and ongoing infections to arthritis. Almost without exception these complaints clear up when wheat is excluded from the diet. You can use a detox plan as a bit of a cold, sharp shock – using it to give up wheat, and then returning to a diet that is wheat-free afterwards. There is a wide range of other grains available, including buckwheat (different family), rice, oats, quinoa, amaranth and corn.

Hand in hand with wheat are cow's produce or dairy foods. Again our consumption of them is often too high for health – we can put milk on our morning cereal, have it in tea, spread butter or some cheese on toast – all before we leave the house in the morning, and so it continues through the day. Cow's dairy food is another prime suspect in all mucus conditions, and is also associated with digestive complaints from indigestion to diarrhoea. Giving it up for a short time is wholly beneficial, and cow's dairy produce is eliminated from all the detox plans in this book. If like wheat you can wean yourself off it while following your detox plan and not return it to your normal everyday diet, your health would be sure to benefit. Needs for calcium can be adequately met while following a detox by the inclusion of small amounts of goat's and sheep's products which do not seem to cause the same health challenges. A wide range of vegetables and herbs also provide calcium, so a varied diet is once again the best answer in the long term.

Drinking lots of good quality, still water while you are

detoxing will enable your system to flush itself fully, and will make life easier on your kidneys. The other drinks are all neutral in their effect – they will not overstimulate or create any further build-up of toxins in the system at a time when you are trying to rid your body of impurities. The herbal teas and juices that are recommended all have specific health benefits. Not drinking enough is one of the easiest mistakes to be made when following a detox plan of any length, and will only impair the profoundly positive effects of all your efforts.

Starting the day, as many of the detox plans do, with a drink of warm water with a slice of lime or lemon will enhance elimination and cleanse the palate. It is a great way to start the day and rinse away some of the impurities that will have collected in the system through the work that your body will have been doing through the night shift.

With such a change to your regular eating plan, you rarely become bored while following a detox. The changes to your taste buds mean that eating becomes a real treat, and you will also start to notice that you become more sensitive – hearing, sight and your sense of touch all become slightly heightened and you are generally likely to feel more alive, and to be more responsive. There is little excuse to break your detox before time, and this is made even easier with the shorter one-, two- and four-day detox plans. A little forward planning will enable you to time it well so as to avoid any potential pitfalls – and that needn't mean locking yourself in for the duration. It is just as easy to order a salad as it is to order a sandwich, or to take a packed lunch with you when you are out or travelling. Most restaurants are only too happy to put together a mixed vegetable or fruit platter, depending on your instructions, and dining out with friends need not be daunting if you offer to bring the salad course. All the efforts that you make in preparation for your detox will enable it to be a complete success.

One of the greatest benefits that comes with every detox is the sense of being more in touch with your body and with its needs. Every time this connection is strengthened, it makes it a little easier to trust your intuition and listen to your body's needs. If you find yourself at the end of your detox plan and don't feel like returning to a full diet, trust your body and follow its lead. Stay with your programme until you feel like eating a wider diet again. You could safely detox for much longer than any of the programmes in this book without any cause for concern, but your body is likely to let you know when it is ready to move on. Once your body has caught up with itself and carried out whatever healing and repair work it needed to, you will find yourself drawn once again to a wider range of foods.

CHAPTER 7

CLEANSING TECHNIQUES

There is a range of simple and easy-to-use techniques that will enhance the effectiveness of your detox, and that can be used at other times for their feel-good factor A prescription for regular doses of fresh air is one of the healthiest things you can possibly take to augment the effectiveness of your detox plan, and to improve your general health – increasing the amount of oxygen that is available to your cells and improving the condition of your heart and lungs, exercising your internal organs and ridding your body of excess carbon dioxide. Breathing techniques are essential to cope with our polluted environment, and also to maximise the benefits of getting lots of good air into the system – essential for the working capacity of the whole body – and helping us detoxify the blood from the effects of carbon dioxide.

These other techniques will re-energise and destress your system. They can form a valuable part of your detox plan, and will also provide a good basis for continuing on the work of regular cleansing once your programme is complete. They are exercises that you can do every day of your life, whether you are actively detoxing or not.

BREATHING WELL

We breathe all the time, and naturally assume we are doing it right, but we could almost all benefit from deeper, more relaxed breathing patterns. A full, easy breath right down into the belly increases oxygen consumption and helps eliminate carbon dioxide from the system more fully, and more quickly. You can do this any time and anywhere. Breathe out all the air from your lungs – let your shoulders collapse forwards a little as you really empty your chest cavity, and then pause for just a moment. When you breathe in again, concentrate on taking the breath right down into your belly in a long, slow, smooth and continuous breath. Push out your abdominal muscles slightly to make room for the full breath. Pause for a moment when you feel full, and then breathe out all the way once again, letting the breath leave your body from this point. Repeat this for a few cycles, and then return to the exercise regularly throughout the day. You will soon notice that you are quite naturally breathing in this way more of the time.

Every time you take a full, deep, easy breath your diaphragm relaxes and then contracts. This rhythmic movement sets up a gentle flowing pressure on all your internal organs in turn, giving them a subtle inner massage that will help with function and the ease with which they are able to work. This movement also helps peristalsis – the way food is moved through the gut – and will support the development of good muscle tone in the abdominal region. Good breathing habits are also of great benefit to the skin, which shares with the lungs the responsibility for exchanges with the air around us. Your skin breathes too, absorbing oxygen and discharging carbon dioxide which has formed in the tissues. Use these breathing exercises in conjunction with skin treats such as body brushing (see page 86) and dry or oil massage (see page 87).

Take a cleansing breath whenever you feel the need to instantly clear your system or your mind, or your emotions: take a deep breath in, as fully and totally as you can, and then pause for a second. Imagine yourself being able to breathe out any disharmony, or toxins, or disease, and let it be carried away, right out of your system on the breath. Breathe out, and see whatever image represents your current difficulty being wafted out of your body and away from you. Take another full, deep, cleansing breath in, and this time see in your mind's eye the fresh air come right into your middle, and then diffuse throughout your body, filling you with fresh, clear energy. Repeat this as often as you need to throughout the day.

DRY SKIN BRUSHING

This is one of the quickest and most effective ways you can benefit your whole body. It makes an invigorating and energising start to the day, and you will see instant results in the softness of your skin and, through the connections between your skin and your lung, bowel and kidney functions, feel considerably lighter and freer with a system that is working better. It all takes just a few minutes a day.

The skin can become clogged with dead cells, and this reduces your ability to eliminate through the skin, and to let your skin 'breathe'. You expel uric acid and other toxins through your skin, along with salt and some nitrogen-containing metabolic waste such as ammonia. When your skin is not functioning well the strain has to be taken up by the body's other eliminative routes and organs. Giving your skin a boost like this will greatly relieve, and may even resolve, any mucus conditions such as sinus troubles and congestion.

Regular skin brushing also stimulates your lymphatic system – the body's waste collection service. This collects refuse from the cells and transports it out of the area and into treatment centres (lymph nodes) where it can be processed and neutralised. These are the areas or glands in your neck that become swollen when you are fighting a cold, and they are also dotted throughout the body, including major sites in the groin, armpits and upper chest. When you have a cold, or your immune system is fighting a battle against infection, the resultant debris is transported via the lymphatic system to the lymph nodes – and swollen nodes are a sure sign that your body is fighting on the immune front.

Brushing your skin with a natural bristle brush is an important part of any detox plan. Do this at the start of the day before you bathe. Begin working your way up over your entire body, starting on the soles of your feet and working towards your heart. Brush your way up each leg, and up your front and back, then brush your hands and up your arms. Finish by brushing down your neck and across your shoulders, making the strokes in the direction of your heart. (This also directs the lymph towards its largest nodes in the upper chest.)

Use the brush as vigorously as you can – you will be surprised that quite a firm pressure actually feels best, but do not brush over any skin rashes or areas of irritation. Do not skin brush if you suffer with nervous irritation or any major pelvic disturbances.

MASSAGE

Massage can be a perfect complement to any detox programme. Beyond the wonderful sensations and hedonistic pleasure of relaxing and receiving a massage, your body benefits in a host of different ways. Lymphatic drainage is improved, getting a mechanical aid to its waste disposal function; general circulation is improved, and the nervous system receives a very positive stimulation. A visit to a massage therapist is a wonderful aid to your detox, but if this is not possible you can do a lot for yourself, at home.

Dry skin massage requires a light touch which will gently stimulate all the nerve endings in your skin and wake it up. You can do this every morning as your skin takes an air bath – just lightly stroke yourself all over with the flat of your hands; you can reach almost all of your body. Imagine that you are in the shower, only instead of rubbing soap in and having water pouring down over your body, you are just rubbing, and the air is washing you off.

Massage with oils allows you to work a little more deeply on your body and to really get things moving. Choose a nice, nourishing oil such as olive or sunflower and warm it a little by placing on a saucer over a bowl of warm water, or standing it on top of the radiator for a few minutes. Take some of the oil in your hands and rub it in, then let your hands glide over your body, following its contours and finding all its soft, yielding places. You may like to start on a small area – feet are usually very receptive – and then work on to cover more of your body. Add two drops of an essential oil to perfume your massage and bring its own therapeutic benefits. Choose sandalwood to help support your kidneys, geranium for a mood lift, or ylang-ylang for a more sensual tone.

EXERCISE

When you move, you not only aid detoxification through the

mechanical pressures of your movement: you also do positive things by reinforcing your own mind–body link. Your mind gets extra energy in the form of glucose that is carried in the increased blood supply, and all your system benefits. They key to exercising successfully is to find something that you enjoy doing, and then to carry on doing it.

Taking some form of daily exercise is a fundamental part of any detox plan. You can combine it with other non-food essentials, such as getting some fresh air, practising some deep and relaxed breathing, and even having a massage; but you need to get some form of exercise each day.

Weight-bearing exercise is particularly useful because of its beneficial effects on the bones and its ability to help ward off the effects of osteoporosis – the bone-thinning complaint that is so common as oestrogen levels drop after the menopause. Regular weight-bearing exercise can be as simple as walking, dancing, or playing tennis. Or you can find a trampoline, or try fencing, or take a t'ai chi class. Anything you do while bearing your own weight will have a positive effect; but most benefits come from repeated, ongoing exercise of this type, and from quick or sudden movements, such as in dancing, playing netball or tennis, or more active forms of martial art such as judo or ki-aikido.

HYDROTHERAPY

This is the therapeutic use of water, either at temperature or under pressure, or just for its own intrinsic qualities. Think of the pleasure of lying in a Jacuzzi, or of sitting in a steam-bath. Both of these are legitimate 'treats' that will enhance the effects of whatever detox plan you are following. Whenever you enjoy a long soak in the bath, you are experiencing some of the healing power of hydrotherapy. If you add a handful of Epsom salts to your bath water for the long soak, you will encourage your muscles to relax and unwind. Make sure that you rest for at least fifteen minutes afterwards though, because the effects can be quite strong, and top up your fluid levels with another long drink of good-quality water.

Add a few drops of essential oil to your bath water to wake up your senses and stimulate elimination. Rosemary and chestnut are both stimulating for the circulation, clove bud is warming and excellent to chase away mucus concerns, and eucalyptus will cleanse the chest and sinuses and stimulate lymphatic activity.

Use the shower to stimulate circulation and really wake up your system. Switch the spray to cold, or as cool as you can tolerate, and then back to warm a few times to wake up your entire body. Always finish on the coolest setting. You can use this to target specific body parts that could use a bit of stimulation or toning, and this is a very successful way to work with any cellulite.

In the warmer weather, try cold water paddling as part of your morning routine. Do not do this if you experience any menstrual irregularity, but otherwise it is quite a tonic, and is perfect for sluggish or overtaxed systems. It is a very stimulating and refreshing habit that will boost your overall circulation and mean an end to cold feet for ever!

After your morning wash routine, fill the bath with enough cold water to cover your ankles, take a deep breath, and step in. Walk up and down for about 60 steps with each foot. When you step out of the water your feet will feel alive and tingling, and considerably warmer. If you do not have access to a bath you can do this in a large washing-up or other bowl: just be certain to step up and down, transferring all your weight as though you were walking. You can also do this, if you have the opportunity, in the sea – a good excuse for an early morning paddle – or on a patch of clean grass that is wet with early-morning dew.

This easy cold water treatment is a boon to your circulation and a boost for the lymphatic system. It takes advantage of a primitive life-saving function that recognises that your feet are getting colder and radically increases your blood supply to that area in order to keep you warm. When you paddle every day the positive effects are long-lasting, which means improved health throughout your body, and an end to cold feet throughout the winter months.

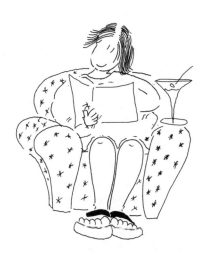

CHAPTER 8

CLEARING YOUR MIND

Your mind and body are intimately connected, even though we often think of them as being quite separate. Every tiny finger movement you make is controlled by a part of your brain. The way you are sitting now is governed partly by your brain sending messages to your postural muscles, and partly by your state of mind.

How we feel is reflected in our posture. When we are depressed our shoulders slump, and movements become heavier and slower. When we are feeling positive and bright we hold our heads higher, move with more of a spring in our step, and have an air of expansiveness and generosity about ourselves.

Our thought processes and overall feelings of wellbeing send messages throughout the body, influencing everything, from the way we stand and move to the way we sleep, our appetite and even our ability to understand and achieve new things.

■ Wake up your mind by seeing if you can change your opinions about things and people, yourself included.

■ Follow a current news story in depth, and see what if feels like to take an opposing view to your usual one.

■ Challenge yourself with new input, and find ways to express your thoughts and ideas.

Keeping a journal is a good way to record your thoughts and dreams; those things that inspire you, and your own inner demons, can all be downloaded on to the page. Journalling is a wonderful way to kick-start your creativity and provides a safe and secure outlet for your own emotions. It can be a great way to begin getting to know yourself better.

We can influence our thoughts positively and consciously to ensure that we are creating the best possible internal atmosphere for ourselves. Too often the things that influence us are beyond our control – the teachings of elders, or parents, or the faith which we grew up in, or even the more widespread impact of society's rules and the advertising that pervades so many aspects of our lives. We can be bombarded with information and PR or sales talk every time we turn on the TV, or walk down the street, or read the paper. Finding out what is true for ourselves can take some time. First we need to sort through the jumble of things we accept as facts, and then decide if they are wholly beneficial and are in fact working for us on an individual level.

As we grow and learn and experience more of life, our store of facts that we hold to be true about the world, and about ourselves, can become overloaded. Sometimes this can cause conflict. If nothing else, it is rather like having a filing system that is bulging at the seams, and doesn't facilitate ease of access to any of our feelings and emotions or our thought processes. Spring-cleaning the mind can be as radical or as perfunctory as you choose.

You can start right away by taking a look at your reactions to things that have happened today, and assess whether they have all expressed your own deepest truths, and whether those truths are your own or have been grafted on from someone else. Review the events of your day, especially your interactions with others, and pay particular attention to any feelings or loose ends that you notice.

Think about the concepts you hold to be true about yourself. Do you consider yourself to be magically wonderful – a unique individual with special gifts? Or is your sense of self a duller image, perhaps more concerned with perceived imperfections, or inadequacies? The things that we hold to be true about ourselves become self-fulfilling prophecies. When we believe that we are capable of greatness, we come closer to achieving it than if we sense that we are doomed to failure. On an everyday level, the little voice that speaks to us from within often speaks with a less-than-encouraging message, highlighting shortcomings, or reinforcing old messages of fear.

We can change the tone of that voice and make sure that the messages we hear are positive, life-affirming and encouraging. The power of positive thought is awesome. It can enable us to feel better about ourselves, and to spread that feeling of goodwill, and to achieve what we strive for, and to become our own heroes and sheroes.

AFFIRMATIONS

An affirmation is a positive intention which you can place in your awareness and allow to grow like a seed, until it bears fruit and takes over from any previous, less focused or less useful thoughts. The beauty of an affirmation is that once you have perfected it and begun using it, it will grow of its own accord. You return to it as often as you like to water and tend it, but the seed continues to grow – the thought itself will do the work.

Target one area of your life to begin with, and identify

something you feel could be changed. This can be anything from your attitude to work to something much more personal, such as your ease in communicating, or the way you use food to hide your emotions. Say to yourself right now all the statements that you believe to be true about yourself and about you in relation to this issue. Write them down, or record them, and apply yourself to finding a way to change your attitude to one that would be more beneficial. The affirmation is the shortest, most apt and precise essence of that change that you can fit into one sentence.

Affirmations work best when they are short and to the point. They need to be positive and forward-looking, and it helps if they are as personal to you as possible. Other things that can be useful are rhyme, which tends to help ideas stick, and the metre of the sentence, so that it sounds and scans well. Good examples of affirmations are: 'I am enough, I have enough, I do enough.' 'I am always in the right place at the right time.' 'Today's the day I ...'

Once you have decided on your affirmation, begin using it as often as you can. Write it down, just to see yourself writing it, and then read it out loud, just to hear yourself say it. Put it on Post-it notes so that you will come across it whenever you look in your desk, or your diary, or open a drawer. Say it in your mind, to yourself, whenever you have a free moment.

Return to your project and review the affirmation every week. See whether it is still the most appropriate thing for you to be saying to yourself ; over time you will find that new ideas have come to you, and you may have noticed some shifts in your stance on the issue. Reflect this is in your new affirmation for the following week.

VISUALISATIONS

This is a great way to harness the strength of our imagination and use it to support our own best efforts. It is a formalised way to daydream, and is something we can all do. Whether you prefer to set the stage and watch a film roll inside your head, or just to capture still images in your mind's eye, the use of these will support your intentions. Visualisations can be used very successfully with affirmations to create a really strong energy for change.

You can use this skill to fight infection in your body by picturing armies of immunity overwhelming any invaders, or by 'seeing' a houseful of maids cleaning up any cellular debris, or as rays of warming sunlight reaching in and banishing any cold or darkness throughout your body. Again, the images that you use will be most effective if they are personal to you, so let your imagination roll and see what pictures come to mind. You can also use visualisations to 'see' yourself achieving change out there in the world, from achieving success in a job interview to handling confrontation more effectively.

Relax before you start your visualisation exercise, and this will make it more effective. Close your eyes, and make sure you are feeling relaxed and comfortable. Take a few easy, deep breaths, and clear your mind of any worries or anxieties. Let the breath carry any physical tensions away too.

You can begin by freely associating – calling to mind a few key words, or the feelings surrounding a particular thing, and see what images come to mind. It can be easier if you picture a screen in front of your eyes for images to be projected onto, or a school board or page of blank paper that pictures can appear on. Experiment until you find what works for you.

Use your visualisation skills regularly to enhance your affirmations and intentions, or on their own to try things out, or experiment with new ways of looking at things and doing things.

MEDITATION

This is an extremely effective way to clear your mind. There is a long tradition of it in Eastern cultures, where it often accompanies other training such as yoga and breathing exercises. These techniques all fit together to bring harmony to our lives.

Practised on its own, meditation can become a valuable oasis of calm within a busy life. There are many different schools that teach different techniques, but they are all reaching towards the same goal, which is the attainment of inner calm or peace and tranquillity. This is achieved in part through the absence of thought. In practice, this means using focusing techniques to still your conscious mind and stop the seemingly endless flow of thoughts that flood through it.

The actual experience of meditation is different from person to person. Some experience it as a quiet time when the freedom from restless thought patterns allows replenishment and a sense of rejuvenation. It is also a time when intuition can surface, and can lead to blissful or peak experiences when one feels in contact with something greater than ourselves. A regular practice can lead to feelings of improved alertness, and a general sense of being refreshed and centred or grounded.

Early morning is a great time to meditate, and you can also make some time for it at the end of the day – so your wakefulness is sandwiched between two periods of intense stillness, calm and clarity. Aim to spend about 20 minutes for each meditation, and as you relax into it you will find you settle into your own sense of timing.

You can focus your eyes on a candle flame, or on a clear image that you will retain in your mind's eye when you then close your eyes; or you can try repeating a gentle humming sound, or a mantra. This is a special, meaningful word that will help focus your attention. You can choose your own – something that is very precious to you such as 'love' or 'peace'.

A lovely way to meditate is to work with your attention – becoming mindful of what you pay attention to – and then moving that attention to the centre of yourself, where you can pay attention to the stillness and calm that is there. Do this by settling yourself in a comfortable position, and closing your eyes. Notice the sounds that you can hear around you, and any aromas that you can sense. Become aware of the feeling of sitting in that position, and then of the sensations of support from your chair or cushion, and the feel of the fabric of your clothes on your skin. Notice how your body moves even when you are sitting quite still. It moves in response to your breathing. Take a moment to focus on your breath – the sensation you feel on your upper lip as you breathe in and out and the air touches you there. Take your awareness inside yourself then, as you notice the ebb and flow of your breathing and its slow, gentle and rhythmic patterns. Linger there, and just stay with the feelings and sensations, the awareness of what is going on, rather than any mental thoughts or ideas you may have about it.

There are many ways to meditate and they do not all involve sitting still and focusing your attention inwards. Some exercise forms such as yoga and t'ai chi are known as moving meditations, because they can be performed in a meditative way and can become part of a meditation practice.

Once you can access this still centre, you can use your intention to make sure that more of your time is spent in this way; anything you do can be done in a meditative way, or become part of a meditation. Preparing food can become a part of your meditation if you place your attention on everything you are doing – attend to the vegetables as you choose them, pick them up, clean them, slice them and add them to your dish. Eating can become part of your meditation, when you confirm your intention to nourish yourself spiritually as well as physically with each meal.

CHAPTER 9

NO TIME TO DETOX

Even if you cannot devote one full day to a detox plan, you can still support your body's own best efforts and make sure that its eliminative work is continuous and successful. There are some basic things that you can add to your daily routine to make sure that your body's work is as easy as possible, and that you are making space for some cleansing.

Choosing foods that have been naturally rather than chemically grown means that you are making life simpler for your body, and reducing the workload for your liver – which in turn means you are likely to have more energy, and to experience fewer toxic headaches.

Eating seasonally helps keep your body in sync with the world that is right outside your window, and will go a long way towards ensuring that you are getting all the natural elements that you need to keep yourself in full health and with maximum energy.

Simply making sure that you enjoy your meals, and that you chew them well, will make an enormous impact upon your health. You cannot digest your food well if you are stressed, so the better your company – even if it's your own – and the more restful or beneficial your surroundings, the easier you make the work for your body. Carbohydrate digestion begins in your mouth and ends in your stomach, so your best chance to ensure maximum energy and savour the taste of what you eat is to chew your food as well as you can.

Specific Choices

Your own food choices can help your body cleanse itself. All cruciferous vegetables (where the leaves grow in a cross), e.g. broccoli, cauliflower, kale, and cabbage are very good. They are packed with helpful enzymes and will support the liver in its own best efforts of detoxification. The bitter herbs and vegetables also stimulate the liver, so add a small handful of young nettle leaves to spring soups and salads, or choose to start a meal with a little green salad, add some chicory or endive, or take a little Swedish Bitters (see page 29) before your meal. Raw beetroot should also be on your list of foods to grate into a salad as a regular treat for your liver.

Eating Out

This doesn't mean you can't still benefit from a no-time detox ... make some careful choices in terms of where you are eating, and be selective with the menu choices you face.

- Choose clear soup rather than a thickened or cream soup, and consider having it as a main course.

- Choose a mixed salad dressed with olive oil and lemon juice. Ask for this as a main course and the kitchen is likely to add an attractive and tasty mix of ingredients.

- Always choose olive oil and lemon juice, or a vinaigrette or French dressing, rather than mayonnaise.

- Pick a mixed-grain roll rather than a baguette, or skip the bread altogether.

- Choose stir-fried, grilled, baked or steamed foods over fried.

■ Choose plain dishes rather than those with a sauce or gravy.

Ask for a vegetable platter as a main course, and you will often get a delicious selection to make a healthy meal with a salad.

At Home

Make good, cleansing choices when you are shopping, so that there are always some good detox-supporting foods at home. Make sure you have a full fruit bowl, and keep salads and other vegetables in the fridge and ready for making a quick snack. If you are tempted to pick on savoury foods, make a dish of crudités and keep them with a healthy dip. Those with a sweet tooth will find few things sweeter than fresh grapes, or a slice of pineapple.

Keep salt off the table and you will notice a dramatic change in the way your body works. This can reduce your salt intake substantially, and really encourage the natural detoxification that your kidneys do. It will also get rid of any water retention, and will help your taste buds perk up too. Make sure that food is still flavour-packed by adding herbs and spices to your meals, and letting the natural flavour of good foods speak for itself.

A Cleansing Breakfast

In the warmer weather, choose fruit for breakfast. This enables your body to get on with its work of elimination, while making sure that you have the energy that you need to get on with your day. It also introduces some plant fibre (especially if you can eat the skins) and a mega-dose of necessary vitamins and some minerals. Choose whatever is seasonally available, and whatever your taste buds draw you to. Endeavour to have some variety, so have a selection of fruits, or choose differently each time you shop.

In the colder weather, you can still benefit from the energy boost, and the rest to digestion, by choosing stewed fruits, or a warmed and soaked compote of dried fruits. Stewed apple that is warmed with a little cinnamon or a clove, and sweetened just before serving with a very little honey or blackstrap molasses, makes a wonderfully warming and soothing breakfast dish that is especially good at easing digestion and facilitating a healthy bowel. Add some blackberries just before the end of cooking, or other berries in autumn for a seasonal treat. Choose any of a host of dried fruits and soak them the evening before; then warm in a saucepan for a nutritious and tasty breakfast alternative.

Skip an Occasional Meal

Substitute a freshly extracted juice in the summer, or a bowl of clear soup or thin porridge in the colder weather, and experience a real energy lift. Pick from the one-day juice cleanse on page 41, or the clear soup listed on page 51, or pick your own blends and ingredients based on the guidelines. This is a great way to keep your energy levels high, whilst giving your body something very simple to do by way of digestion, and enabling it to divert some additional energy towards cleansing.

You can do this as regularly as three or four times a week and feel the benefits. Make sure that you don't just skip the meal and have nothing, though, or you reset your body into fasting mode and risk creating some internal stress and confusion.

Healthy Options

Make the following substitutions to make sure that you are making life as easy and simple as possible for your system, and letting it detox itself naturally. Start slowly by making the substitutions when you are shopping, and you will notice the gradual change translates to genuine health improvements.

CHOOSE	NOT
Herbs and spices	salt
Olive oil and lemon juice	mayonnaise
Fresh fruit	sweets
Olive oil	butter or margarine
Herbal teas and green tea	tea
Dandelion coffee and root blends	coffee
Fresh juices	colas and fizzy drinks
Still water	fizzy water and fizzy drinks
Fresh foods	dried, frozen or canned
Fresh foods	ready meals
Soya alternative to milk	cow's milk
Goat's and sheep's cheeses	cow's cheese
Soya yoghurts	cow's yoghurt
Barley, quinoa, rice, amaranth	wheat

You can harness other natural elements such as the electromagnetics of a Bioflow to reinforce the work of your detox. (See page 115.)

And Finally...

It's not just about foods and choosing them wisely, or when you eat them. Take a moment right now to take in a full, deep, cleansing breath and imagine that as you breathe out you can blow away any tension from your system. Take another full, deep, cleansing breath, and imagine as you breathe out that you are ridding your body of any impurities or unwanteds. Take a last big, deep breath and feel yourself being re-energised, and then breathe out any negative thoughts and feelings.

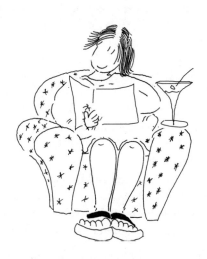

CHAPTER 10

DETOX YOUR LIFE

Why not change the energy around you while you are in the process of changing your inner energy? You can use the vitality and renewed energy you feel from following a detox plan to help you clear out any area of your life from any clutter or unwanteds that might be impeding your progress, or blocking your happiness.

A PERSONAL AUDIT

Clear space is space that is ready and welcoming to new things, so take another look at your home, your work life, your relationships and your sense of self, and see whether the following techniques might help you make some space for new things there.

Take an audit of your day; look at how you spend your time and how you relate to those around you. Note down the benefits you receive from each interaction and how successful you are in all your undertakings. Rate yourself for confidence and self-assurance, as well as for how satisfied you feel with each aspect of your day. Do this every day for one week and then review it to see just what you spend your time on, and what your life comprises. You may uncover a few surprises. You will most certainly be able to identify those times and interactions which are not wholly beneficial or supportive for you right now, and you may have found some situations or challenges, or people, that are positively toxic.

Some things or relationships or scenarios may have run their course, and you might simply be ready to move on to another stage in your life.

Once you have identified some things which are not wholly beneficial to you, you can start to cleanse your life of them by eliminating them from your world. You can do this little by little – a day at a time – or in one concerted effort to revitalise and re-energise your daily life. You can work to eliminate absolutely anything that doesn't serve your ongoing wellbeing and happiness – from meetings with a disagreeable neighbour to being in a job that doesn't satisfy you. The double benefit of doing something about what is no longer needed in your life is that you then develop some time or space in which to do something that *does* further your own goals.

PRACTICAL STEPS

You can use this spirit of detox to eliminate clutter from your home and from your workplace. Feng Shui is a way of studying the energy that flows within and around us, and making sure that it is beneficial to us. It is concerned with the appropriate placement of things, and is very much to do with eliminating anything unnecessary from your physical world.

To apply some basic Feng Shui principles to your situation, think of a breeze or a stream of water flowing into and around the area you are assessing. Would it be able to flow freely? Is the area balanced – would it move too quickly through and out of the area, or are there any places where it could not travel? You can look at your whole home from this point of view, applying it one room at a time, or use it to reorganise your desk.

Getting rid of anything that you don't really use or benefit from gives you a chance to improve the energy flow through your world, and is also an opportunity to continue the work of elimination and carry detox energy into your daily life on another level. When you throw out things that no longer serve you, you make room for positive new influences.

Make a grid for yourself based on the one shown below, and use it to make sure that each aspect of your life is represented in some good and clear way in the area that you are looking to rebalance. Make sure that your point of entry (where you sit if you are using this for your desk, or the door if you are applying this to a room) is somewhere on the bottom line.

Beneficial influences	Inspiration	Partnerships and unions
Inherited influences	Health	Creativity
Unity and wholeness	Career/way in the world	Guardians/ protection

You might like to keep the centre area clear to represent clear, good health; or focus on placing pairs of things in the area of partnerships; or have a blooming plant in your sphere of beneficial influences. There are many ways you can work with this, including moving your furniture around to make the most of each sphere of influence. Placing your bed in the area of creativity might be a good move if you are seeking to conceive, and the area of protection might be a good place to hang a talisman or object of personal significance. These quadrants also correspond with the elements and cardinal directions, and you can explore these connections; or simply concentrate on keeping your clutter out of your career area, and making sure that too much dust doesn't ever settle in the lake of your creativity; or that you always keep your place of inspiration clear and tidy.

There are other practical steps you can take to make sure that your life is as clear and that your energy is flowing as smoothly as it needs to for you to live effectively. Keeping your life in balance is easier once you have done your initial audit, and seen how you spend your time. When you work out what is important to you, it is much easier to apportion your time appropriately and productively. Consider dividing each day into three, and spending eight hours on work, eight hours in play or leisure, and eight hours on yourself. Much of this eight hours would be spent asleep – sleep is something we can never really seem to get enough of, and it is a wonderful complement to any type of detox plan you might be implementing. When we sleep we allow the body's own self-regenerating and healing free rein, and everything from the production of growth hormone to the quality of our skin benefits from getting just an extra hour a night. When we are regularly getting enough sleep it enables us to be much more effective in our waking life.

NEW THINGS

Trying something new is a good way to bring new energy into your world. This can be anything from going salsa dancing to trying a kick-boxing class. Exercise is so good for you on so many different levels, but it is not the only way to bring something new into your life. The energy of detox is about rest and renewal, and just having a day off when you can relax and switch off from ongoing concerns can be remarkably regenerative. Make relaxation time a priority, and maximise its benefits by practising a breathing technique to re-energise your whole body; or do some gentle stretches; or read a book; or just enjoy doing nothing in particular and being free from a timetable, for however short a time. Work out what works for you, and make time for it.

Remember to treat yourself – schedule more time for yourself and the things that you know replenish you. Go for a massage or visit a spa for the day when you can; but when time or funds are short, remember the other things that will give you a lift – like buying yourself flowers, going for a long walk, or just spending some time on your own with your own thoughts and feelings.

Nature provides a wealth of resources to enhance our experience, and flowers have a wonderful role to play – giving such beauty for us to marvel at, and providing the headiest perfumes. They can also be used as remedies in a gentle and effective way to rebalance the subtler system. This can prove a lovely complement to the more instant effects of a physical detox plan, bringing a subtler quality to your programme, and ensuring that your whole energetic system is cleansed and cleared.

Flower remedies are made by capturing some of the essence of the flower and 'potentising' it. This is then preserved and usually bottled, for use whenever we need it. Each flower and blend of flower essences will have a different effect on the system, and an affinity with different parts of your experience. Some especially useful ones to try whilst following any length of detox are from the Dr Bach range, made using European flowers. It is good to use remedies that are locally grown, but follow your intuition with this and if you feel yourself drawn to more exotic ranges, then follow that cue. Crab apple has a strong connection with cleansing and is useful for ridding us of old, worn-out emotions. Olive is useful when there is tiredness, either as your reason for detoxing or when you have been following one of the longer programmes for a week or a month. Holly can help get rid some of the more difficult feelings associated with stagnant energy and it usually proves effective very quickly.

To take flower remedies, put a few drops in a small glass of water and sip. Take at least three times a day, and especially on waking and before you go to bed. You can add several drops to a small bottle of mineral water and sip it through the day; this is especially useful if you are away from home. You can mix up to half a dozen different flower remedies together and take them, and one of the most popular and successful ranges is Dr Bach's Rescue Remedy, which is a blend of flower essences specifically geared for dealing with any kind of shock or stress. It is very good to take if ever you feel stuck in your detox plan, and that things are just not progressing.

When you gather together a range of different aids and techniques to support your efforts, you can maximise the effects of a detox in your life. Just widening your awareness or making it your intention to detox your *life*, and not just your body, opens up a whole new world of possibilities. The more ways you manifest your intentions, and the more levels on which you make your detox effective, the greater your increase in wellbeing and the more energy you will have. It is also an awesome thing when everything you do is geared towards your own positive progress and greater health; it places you in a very powerful position in your own life.

RESOURCES

FURTHER READING

Dylana Accolla with Peter Yates, *Back to Balance*, Newleaf, 1996

Betty Balcombe, *As I See It*, Piatkus, 1995

Kitty Campion, *Handbook of Herbal Health*, Macdonald Sphere, 1985

Deepak Chopra, *Perfect Health*, Bantam, 1990

Oliver and Michele Cowmeadow, *Yin Yang Cookbook*, Optima, 1988

Kenneth Meadows, *Earth Medicine*, Element, 1989

Arabella Morningstar, *The Ayurvedic Cookbook*, Lotus Press, 1990

Stephen Roet, *All in the Mind*, Optima, 1989

Belinda Grant Viagas, *A–Z of Natural Healthcare*, Newleaf, 1997

Belinda Grant Viagas, *Natural Healthcare for Women*, Newleaf, 1997

Belinda Grant Viagas, *Nature Cure*, Newleaf, 1999

FINDING A PRACTITIONER

The information in this book is sufficient for you to undertake your own detox programme. If you have any specific health concerns, or feel the need for individual support, or if this has whetted your appetite for finding out more about natural ways to support your own health, you will need to contact a natural healthcare practitioner or Naturopath. Details of how to contact the author appear below.

When choosing a practitioner, always remember to follow your own judgement and make sure you feel comfortable with them. Ask about their training and any areas of expertise or special interest, but check too how easy you find it to talk to them, and whether you can establish a rapport. It is worth taking time to find the right person who will knowledgeably support and encourage you with their professional advice, experience and care.

CONTACTS

UK
British Complementary Medicine Association
33 Imperial Square
Cheltenham
Gloucestershire GL50 1QZ
fax: 01242 227765
www.bcma.co.uk

Council for Complementary and Alternative Medicine
Park House
206–208 Latimer Road
London W10 6RE
tel: 020 8968 3862
www.rccm.org.uk

Lamberts Nutritional Supplies
1 Lamberts Road
Tunbridge Wells
Kent TN2 3EQ
Tel: 01892 552121

FSC Supplements
Europa Park
Stoneclough Road
Radcliffe
Manchester M26 1GG
tel. 01204 707420

IRELAND
Irish Association of Holistic Medicine
9–11 Grafton Street
Dublin 2
tel. 01 6712788

Naturalife Health Ltd
7 Charvey Court
Rathnew
Co. Wicklow
tel. 0404 62444
www.naturalife.ie

AUSTRALIA
Australian Complementary Health Association
247 Flinders Lane
Melbourne 3000
Victoria
www.vicnet.net.au

Australian Institute of Holistic Medicine
862 North Lake Road
Jandakot
WA 6164
www.waihm.wa.edu.au

Australian Natural Therapists Association
PO Box 856
Coloundra
QLD 4551
www.anta.com.au/

NEW ZEALAND

New Zealand Register of Complementary Health Practitioners
C/o New Zealand Health Network
PO Box 337
Christchurch

Association of Natural Therapies
81 Forrest Hill Road
Milford
Auckland

Society of Naturopaths
Box 19183
Auckland 7
www.naturopath.org.nz/

NORTH AMERICA

America Holistic Health Association
PO Box 17400
Anaheim
CA 92817–7400
www.ahha.org

To contact the author for details of her postal Advice Service, or news about her training courses and workshops, or for a Bioflow electromagnetic product, please write to her at:

PO Box 13386
London NW3 2ZE
or e-mail at: Belindasres@hotmail.com